BE YOUR OWN DOCTOR WITH A[...]

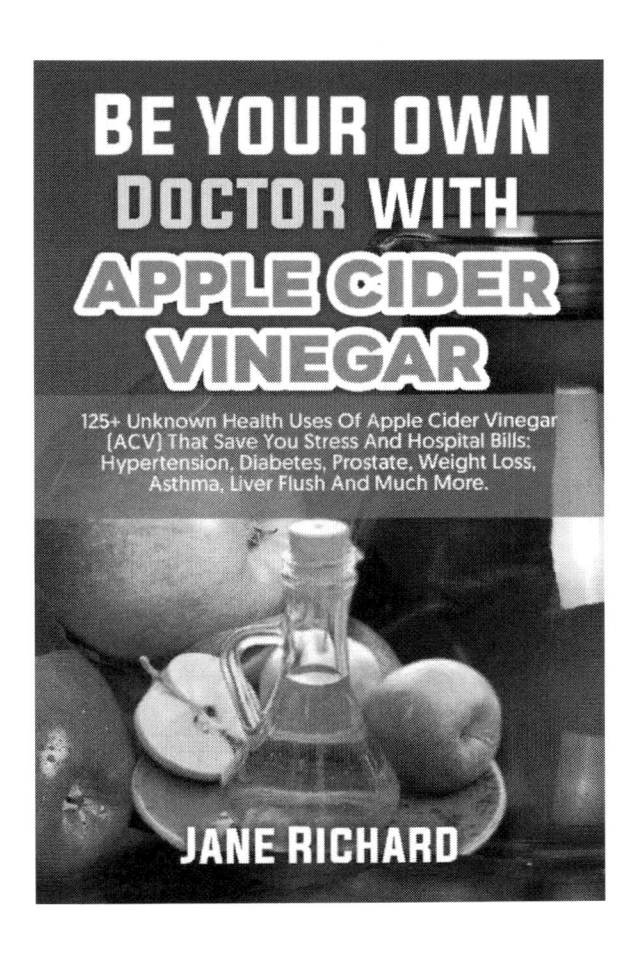

(125+ Unknown Health Uses Of A[...]
That Save You Stress And Hospital Bills: Hyp[...]
Diabetes, Prostate, Weight Loss, Asthma, Liver Flush And
Much More.)

BE YOUR OWN DOCTOR WITH APPLE CIDER VINEGAR

125+ Unknown Health Uses Of Apple Cider Vinegar (ACV) That Save You Stress And Hospital Bills: Hypertension, Diabetes, Prostate, Weight Loss, Asthma, Liver Flush And Much More.

JANE RICHARD

©COPYRIGHT

All Rights Reserved. Contents of this book may not be reproduced in any way or by any means without written consent of the publisher, with exception of brief excerpts in critical reviews and articles.

DEDICATION

This book is dedicated to all persons striving to make the world a better place. Those who labour to leave the word better than they met it.

ACCEPTANCE OF RESPONSIBILITY

We do not lay claim to any perfection, nobody is. Consequently, we accept full responsibility for any deficiency readers might find in this work.

We will cheerfully receive any suggestions to improve on this.

PROLOGUE

'Naturalists believe that, if you were to select just two substances for your family that have usefulnesses and practicability, they would be vinegar and Hydrogen Peroxide. I will add Baking Soda to make three.'

Contents

©COPYRIGHT 2
DEDICATION 3
ACCEPTANCE OF RESPONSIBILITY 4
PROLOGUE 5
SPECIAL NOTICE. 13
DESCRIPTION 14
INTRODUCTION. 18
HISTORY OF VINEGAR. 21
    1.   In Greece Civilisation 22
    2. The Romans Time. 22
    3. The Middle Ages. 23
    4. Vinegar And The Plague 24
    5. Vinegar Of The Four Thieves. 24
    6. Cholera and Vinegar. 25
APPLE CIDER VINEGAR AND HER SISTERS. 26
TYPES OF VINEGAR. 29
    Apple Cider Vinegar. 29
    Balsamic vinegar 29
    Malt vinegar 29
    Rice vinegar 30
    White vinegar. 30
    Wine vinegar, ... 30
DIFFERENCES BETWEEN APPLE CIDER VINEGAR AND WHITE VINEGAR. 32
DOCTORS, DO THEY ALWAYS TELL US THE WHOLE TRUTH? ..35

SIX DON'TS WITH APPLE CIDER VINEGAR. 41
    1. Never Drink ACV Straight. 42
    2. Little At A Time, At The Beginning. 42
    3. On The Skin, Do A Patch Test First. 42
    4. Don't Mix With Other Strong Chemicals. 43
    5. Hydrogen Peroxide. 43
    6. Daily Ingestion. 43
THE USES OF ACV 44
    1. Acid Reflux: Very Discomforting. 44
    2. Acne Astringent: Not Ok For Your Face. 47
    3. Age Spots And Wrinkles: Remove Them. 48
    4. Ageing: Reverse Your Age. 48
    4. Allergies: Stop Them. 49
    5. Amino Acids: You Need Them. 50
    6. Antibacterial Properties: Bacteria In Serious Trouble 51
    7. Antifungal Properties: Kill The Fungi. 52
    8. Appetite: Eat Less, Less Fatty. 53
    9. Artery Plaque Can Kill: Clear The Road For Blood 53
    10. Asthma: Get Clear Airways. 54
    11. Athletes Foot: Wipe It Off. 55
    13. Backache: Straighten Up. 56
    14. Bacterial Cystitis: Clear The Tract. 57
    15. Bedwetting: Too Bad, Stop It. 58
    16. Bites: Soothe The Pains. 59
    17. Bleeding: Stop The Flow 59

18. Blood Sugar: High Sugar, Big Problem. 59

19. Bronchitis: Clear The Mucus. 60

20. Burns: Any Type Of Burns. 61

21. Calcium and Potassium Absorption: So, So Important. 62

22. Cancer: Not Your Friend. 63

23. Cataracts: You Need Good Sight. 64

24. Cellulite: Ugly Fats. 65

25. Cervical Cancer: Do A Dirt Cheap Test. 66

26. Chickenpox: An Enemy of The Skin. 66

27. Cholesterol and Triglycerides: Cut Them Down. 67

28. Conjunctivitis or Pink Eye: Get White Eyeballs. 68

29. Cough: Clear It Off. 69

30. Constipation: Too much Food, Too Much Junk. 70

31. Corns & Calluses: Ugly On Your Toes. 71

32. Cradle Cap Cure: Give The Little One a Smooth Head. 72

33. Dandruff: Clear Off Ugly White Flakes. 72

34. Denture: Happy for A Good Soak. 73

35. Deodorant: Why Not Make Your Own. 74

36. Detoxification: Get The Toxins Out. 75

37. Diabetes: Balance Your Sugar Level. 76

38. Diaper Rashes: Smoothen Baby's Skin. 78

39. Diarrhoea: Stop The Flow. 79

40. Dog Ticks: Dogs Don't Like Them. 80

41. Douching: Keep Female Down Clean And Fresh. 80

42. Dry Hair: Make Hairs Lush Again. 81

43. Ear Drops: Clean The Cochlea Dirt. 81

44. Eczema: Embarrassing. 81

45. Emphysema: Clear The Air Sacs. 83

46. Face Toning: Lighter Face Shines Better. 84

47. Fasting: Body Cleanser. 85

48. Fever Blisters: Ugly Sight, You Don't Want Them. 86

49. Fever: Weakens You, Fight It. 86

50. Fibres: You Also Need Them. 87

51. Flatulence: Ease off the Gas. 88

52. Fleas Spray: Nuisance Fleas. 89

53. Food Poisoning: Uncomfortable. 89

54. Gallbladder: Be Nice to The Flusher. 89

55. Gerd. 90

56. Gingivitis: Protect Your Teeth. 91

57. Hair Conditioner: Easy To Make. 91

58. Hair Follicle Growth: Possible. 92

59. Hair Frizz: Tame Them. 92

60. Hair Rinse. 92

61. Hair: Shine Your Hair. 93

62. Hard water: Remove The Minerals Build-Up. 93

63. Head Ache And Migraines: Signs Of Deeper Trouble? 94

64. Heartburn: Fire In The Thoracic Cavity. 95

65. Hiccups: You Don't Need Them. 95

66. Haemorrhoids: Stop It In Its Track. 96

67. Herpes Virus: Trouble for Virus. 97

68. Hives: Get Relief. 97
69. Hypertension: You Can Avoid It. 98
70. Immunity Booster: Spike Your Immunity. 99
71. Infections: Stop Them in Their Track. 102
72. Inflammation: Not Good Anywhere. 103
73. Inner Ecosystem Balancing: Moving Toward Equilibrium....... 104
74. Insomnia: Sleeping Is Your Right. 104
75. Interstitial Cystitis: Flay The Cramps and Pains. 105
76. Iron absorption: Iron for Strength.................................. 106
77. Irritable Bowel syndrome: Discomforting. 106
78. Joint Pain: Watch It. 107
79. Kidney: Clean The Body's Second Most Important Factory....107
80. Laryngitis: Let's Get Melodious. 108
81. Leg cramps: Free The Legs... 109
82. Lice: Frustrating Scratching In The Public 109
83. Listerine Foot Bath: Clear Off The Dead Cells. 110
84. Liver, Hepatitis: Caring For The Body's First Giant Factory. 111
85. Malnutrition: Beef Up A Little. 112
86. Mentally Handicapped: They Could Be Helped. 114
87. Morning sickness: Sign Of Bundle Of Joy. 114
88. Morning Smoothes: Best Way To Take Off. 115
89. Muscle Stiffness: Supple Muscles Work Best. 116
90. Nail Fungus: Kill Them. 118
91. Nasal Wash: For Free Nasal Passage........................... 119
92. Nausea And Vomiting: Irritating............................... 120

93.	Nerve Pains (Sciatic Nerve Pain): Free The Nerves.	121
94.	Nosebleeds: Embarrassment In The Public.	122
95.	Obesity: Burn Off the Fat.	122
96.	Parasitic Infections: Stop Them.	124
97.	Pest Repellent: Keep The Fleas Away.	125
98.	Parasite & Bug Repelling Body Rinse.	125
99.	Pimples: Hate Them, Confidence Destroyer.	126
100.	Poop (Feces Or Faeces): Clear The Bowels.	126
101.	Porosity: Block The Holes.	127
102.	Healthy scalp: Home to Your Hairs.	127
103.	pH Balance: Balance Your Scalp PH.	128
104.	Prostate: Don't Allow Them to Enlarge.	128
105.	Proriasis: A Smooth Skin Is The Best.	129
106.	Reflexology; Helps With Arthritis.	130
107.	Rheumatoid Arthritis: Could Be Painful.	130
108.	Scurvy.	131
109.	Senility: Sufferers Could Be Helped.	132
110.	Shampoo: Make Your Own.	133
111.	Shingles: Chicken Pox's Sister.	133
112.	Sinuses: Disappears In No Time.	135
113.	Skin Exfoliate: Dead Cells In Trouble.	136
114.	Sore Throat: Pharyngitis, Laryngitis Brother.	137
115.	Sunburn: Summer Sun.	138
116.	Swimmers Ear: Water in the Ear.	139
117.	Teeth: White Teeth Give You Advantage.	140

118. Thirst Quencher: A Summer Need. 141

119. Thrush: A Yeast Infection...142

120. Tiredness: Normal, Now Get Your Strength Back. 142

121. Ulcers: Don't Do It...143

122. Underweight: Flesh Up A Bit. 143

123. Varicose Veins: Ugly Sight..144

124. Vegetarians And Vegans: You Need Apple Cider Vinegar....146

125. Warts: No Need To Scrape...147

126. Weight Loss: Fat Fatty. 147

127. Yeast infection..148

128. Yellow Nails: Make Them white...149

OTHER BOOKS BY THE AUTHOR. 150

ABOUT THE AUTHOR 151

LUCKY YOU, SO SIGN UP FOR A FREE GIVEAWAY 152

WRITE A REVIEW 153

ACKNOWLEDGMENT 155

SPECIAL NOTICE.

Readers may find that both American and British spellings are used in this book. For instance, readers may see color in some places and colour in other places.

You may see fiber and fibre, liter and litre, vapor and vapour, vigour and vigor etc. We crave your indulgence to accept as correct both American and British spellings.

ACV in this book means organic, raw Apple Cider vinegar with the mother and not commercial kinds of vinegar which have no health values. Wherever you see ACV or Vinegar, please read Apple Cider Vinegar.

Organic ACV is brownish in color with the tiny, cobweb "mother" floating in it at the bottom.

This appearance is not eye-friendly, it is non-appealing and so manufacturers went to their labs and gave consumers what they wanted, distilled white vinegar which is medically worthless.

DESCRIPTION.

Apple Cider Vinegar, God's Greatest Gift to Man.

'If you were to select just two substances for your family that have usefulnesses and practicability, they would be Apple Cider Vinegar and Hydrogen Peroxide'

That is the verdict of most Naturalists, only that I will add Baking Soda to make three.

But for usefulnesses, the other two combined cannot hold a candle to Vinegar's face.

For Health assists, Vinegar had been in use for over 10,000 years, which places it in a class of her own.

The Greeks, The Romans, The Egyptians all used vinegar extensively.

The father of modern medicine, Hippocrates used vinegar which he prescribed for treating wounds, sores, and tract infection.

Not to forget, the great Roman soldiers also used vinegar to treat wounds, quench thirst on long journeys, and to treat a variety of conditions in their camp.

Christopher Columbus and his men on their voyage to discover America in 1492 had barrels of vinegar to prevent scurvy. U.S. Civil war soldiers did the same.

If Vinegar was useful then, it is even more useful now.

Useful in homes, in the kitchen, on the farm, in the office, in the car, and anywhere.

If you were looking for an all-purpose compound, it is Vinegar. If you were looking for a 'do all' vinegar is it.

And are they many? You bet, but before we go further, I will let you into a secret.

Ok, bring your ear closer to me. I am whispering, 'The Immunity Booster and Detoxification Therapies' in this book fight almost any illness.

If these two are all you learn in this book and put to use, you would have gotten more value than the cost of this book.

And that is just one of the over 120 health issues treated.

From little ailments like diarrhea, sore throat, constipation to more serious health conditions like diabetes, liver flush, thrush, and even cancer.

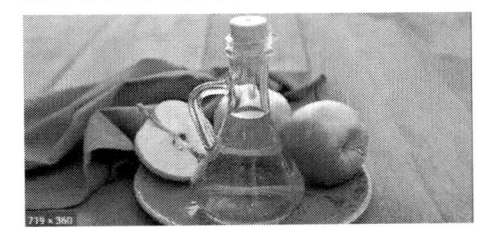

If you live healthily, eat healthily and you own a copy of this book, there will be no need for you to see a doctor or dentist except for hereditary issues.

That reminds me, ACV will make your teeth whiter. How to do that is in this book.

We are not oblivious of the fact that there are countless food recipes with ACV out there, but **'Be Your Own Doctor With Apple Cider Vinegar'** has no food recipes.

However, if you are looking for a book that dwells extensively on essential health remedies to give you a bouncing healthy body through and through, this is the book.

Although I have used Apple Cider Vinegar for diverse purposes, my greatest moment was when I deployed it to fight my daughter's pimples. It was like, Dad where did you keep that since. I became her health hero.

The book handles important health issues in a way that tickles.

A glimpse inside **'Be Your Own Doctor With Apple Cider Vinegar'**.

- Acne Astringent: Not OK For Your Face.
- Artery Plaque Can Kill: Clear Road For Blood.
- Blood Sugar: High Sugar, Big Problem.
- Cataracts: You Need Good Sight.
- Cervical Cancer: Dirt Cheap Test.
- Dog Tick: Dogs Don't Like Them.
- Douching: Keep Female Down Clean And Fresh.
- Hypertension: You Can Avoid It.
- Immunity Booster: Spike Your Immunity.
- Liver, Hepatitis: Caring For The Body's First Giant Factory
- Obesity: Burn Off The fat.
- Rheumatoid Arthritis: Could Be Painful.
- Ulcer: No, no, don't do it. We even tell you what you should not use Apple Cider Vinegar for.

There is a chapter in this book we trust you would like:

'Doctors, Do They Always Tell Us All The Truth'? It will interest you and make you ask questions. For example, is it true that Doctors kill more than guns? The answer is inside the book.

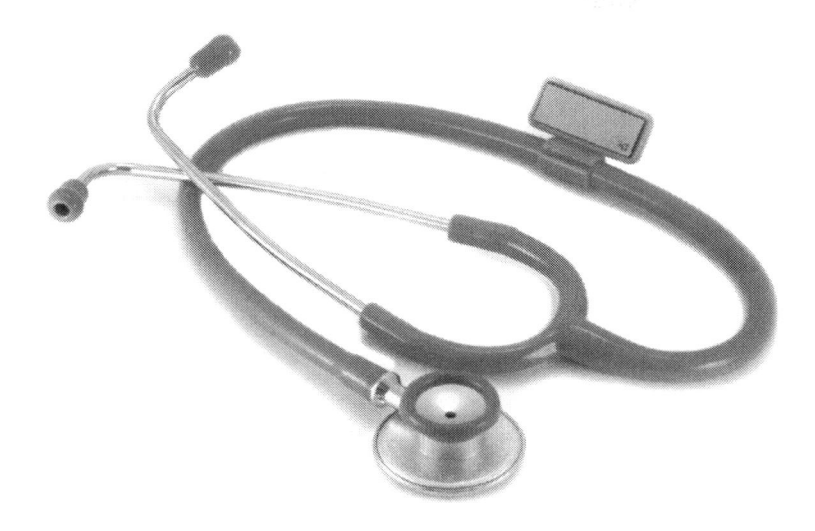

And much more.

One more thing, we arranged the book alphabetically. We do not abandon you in a haze of topics struggling to find your way. Just go to the content and make your pick.

You would like to ask, why is ACV so powerful with multipurpose and diverse applications?

Sometimes, it works in opposite directions, in both ends of a spectrum. For example, while it helps you to put on some flesh, it also helps people with fat to burn it.

The answer really is nobody knows expect to tell you that ACV is packed full with major vitamins, powerful antioxidants, useful acids such as Acetic Acid (a major constituent) and Malic acid, enzymes, fibers, and several minerals, which make it a topmost top-of-the-shelve chemical for home remedies you will ever get out there.

Apple Cider Vinegar is so complex to understand except to say that it is a God's riddle, which is why it is called God's greatest gift to Mankind.

"**Be Your Own Doctor With Apple Cider Vinegar**' explores this gift and exposes to you how you can use it to have a healthier living, saving you stress and hospital bills.

Trust me, as I have found out, owning a copy will add much value to your family and household.

Start living an illness-free life the cheap way by owning a copy of **Be Your Own Doctor With Apple Cider Vinegar** by clicking the buy button at the top before the price goes up. Don't forget to come back here to write a review.

INTRODUCTION.

In recent years, Complementary and Alternative (CAM) healthcare delivery has gained more popularity and acceptability among the populace which has made Naturalists and practitioners research for more uses and applications.

More people are turning to CAM as the cost of orthodox medicine has spiralled out of control and beyond the pockets of average earners.

Converts have not been disappointed as they have, by and large, been having their health needs met by CAM.

In a report, in 1990, about thirty-three percent of Americans had used CAM and by 2002, the figure had doubled.

As things are currently, there are no reasons or signs to suggest that this trend will be reversed. Actually, pointers are that CAM is not prepared to yield to orthodox medicine.

CAM has come to stay and that is a fact that conventional medicine has to contend with.

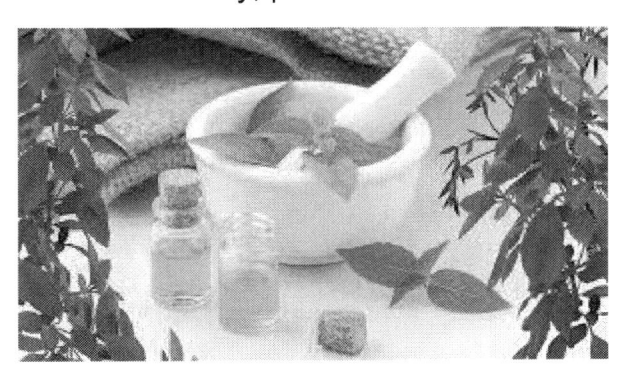

We are happy to announce that, Apple Cider Vinegar, made from apple is with them at the top of Complementary and Alternative (CAM) therapy.

Remember the saying; an apple a day keeps the doctor away. It was true then and even truer now.

Having written '150+ Uses of Baking Soda You Never Knew', I took up the challenge to take a deep look at vinegar, and what I found awed me.

It was immediately clear to me that I could not do justice to hundreds of its uses in a book.

That apart, I thought mixing them together would get readers confused. So it was decided, for this book, to concentrate on the health uses of this great substance called vinegar.

And here is the new baby that decision birthed. **'Be Your Own Doctor With Apple Cider Vinegar'**

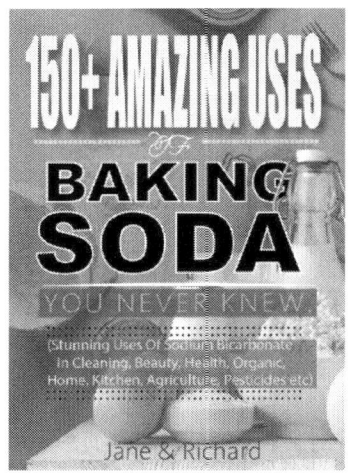

Here is a compound that had been with us for more than ten thousand years.

Vinegar was used by Hippocrates, the father of modern medicine as a prescription to treat wounds, cuts, and other medical conditions.

Christopher Columbus and his men on their voyage to discover America in 1492 had barrels of vinegar for the prevention of scurvy.

During the United States civil war, soldiers used Apple Cider Vinegar for assistance in many areas.

Now, imagine that you can get this invaluable material cheaply and easily which you can store in your fridge for any-time use to become your own doctor? What a privilege.

Agreed that there are OTC products out there doing wonders but at what cost?

Unlike ACV that has no side effects, those proprietary products are costly and most of them solve a problem only to deposit two others.

Skip their pills, run away from their creams, drop their tablets, and have nothing to do with their concoctions.

Get a bottle of Apple Cider Vinegar and this book which you are lucky to have already. That is all you need to give yourself and household good health care.

This book is damn easy to use. Just go to the contents which are arranged alphabetically and pick the ailment disturbing you and go straight to the page. Get the recipe and follow.

It is as simple as that. Be your own Doctor.

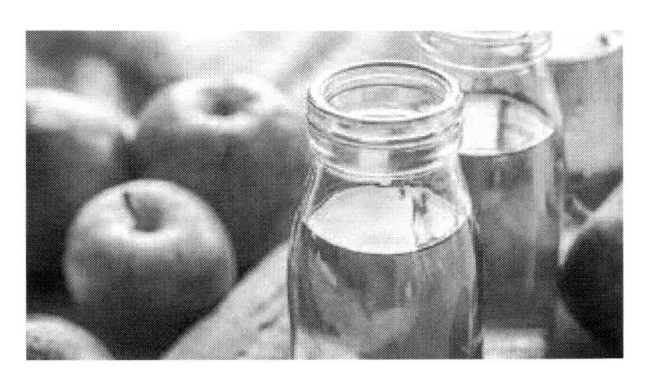

HISTORY OF VINEGAR

Vinegar is as old as History itself with a record dating back to 10,000 years.

It is mentioned in the bible and there are vats of Vinegar in Egypt dating back to years before Pharaoh.

The Egyptians and the Babylonians used Vinegar extensively. Mixed with water, they used vinegar to preserve foods.

They used kinds of vinegar and water to preserve foods when on long journeys while farmers and travellers used the mixture to quench thirst.

Vinegar recorded history dates as far back as around 5000 B.C, starting with the Babylonians and then the Egyptians in 3000 B.C. and the Chinese in 1200 B.C.

Because vinegar kills germs and bacteria, many cultures have found it useful not only for health reasons but also for medicinal, and cleaning uses.

1. In Greece Civilisation.

During the Greek civilization, Vinegar was prominent.

The father of modern medicine, Hippocrates used vinegar which he prescribed for treating wounds, sores, and tract infection.

They consumed a mixture of vinegar, water, and honey which they called oxycrat kept in special vases called Oxydes.

2. The Romans Time.

The Romans had a variety of vinegar recipes from very simple ones to very famous ones.

Apicus, a famous Roman Epicurean gastronomist had several recipes each including vinegar.

His contemporary, Colimella left many vinegar recipes and yeast used to favour fermentation in wine to purify and remove unpleasant odors.

On the cross, the Roman soldiers offered Jesus Christ a mixture of vinegar and gall to drink though as torture rather than a relief. He refused.

This means the people of that time were as familiar with Vinegar as we are today.

They used it to clean, used it as a preservative, used it as an antibiotic, as a condiment, and as a medicine.

During the Roman time, they had many sauces made from vinegar.

They used it as dressing for their 'acetane', to dress meat and vegetable salads served between meals.

They also used it to preserve fish in addition to other several uses that made life more interesting and pleasant for them.

Not to forget, the great Roman soldiers also used vinegar to treat wounds, quench thirst on long journeys, and to treat a variety of conditions in their camp.

Hannibal Barca, a famous Carthaginian general (247-183 B.C.) used Vinegar to break rocks for his soldiers and animals to pass through having made the rocks friable by burning.

3. The Middle Ages.

As said earlier, Christopher Columbus and his men on their voyage to discover America in 1492 had barrels of vinegar for the prevention of scurvy. United States soldiers also used vinegar during the Civil war.

4. Vinegar And The Plague.

During the black plague of the 14th century that killed one out of three in Marceille, Vinegar was used extensively.

Marseille people protected themselves by holding a sponge soaked in Vinegar under their noses without using the mouth to breathe or swallowing saliva.

Nurses who assisted Doctors always had a basin of vinegar in hand where the medics could wash their hands before and after treating patients.

When the plagues subsided, the walls of houses where sick people were, were washed with Vinegar.

5. Vinegar Of The Four Thieves.

Have you heard of Vinegar of the four thieves? During the 1720 plague in Marseille, these four (some say seven) could sack a whole town and get away with it, using bandage soaked with vinegar around the forehead to prevent them from being infected.

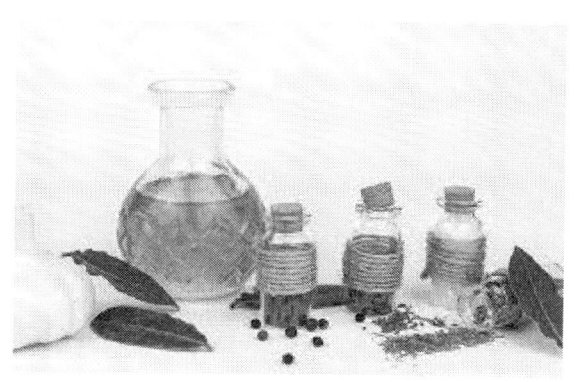

They used vinegar for ablution and gargle, the ingredients not known to many.

They were caught eventually and sentenced to death but their lives were spared because of the same vinegar.

Later a French expert tried to clone their recipe.

6. Cholera and Vinegar.

In very recent years, vinegar is known to be used to treat cholera.

Between 1830 and 1884, the government passed a law that anybody who had visited a sick person must wash their hands in vinegar, know full well that cholera can be transmitted through food.

They were also to wash fruits and vegetables before eating.

Vinegar did prove itself to be an effective disinfectant.

It did then and still does now in addition to many other great uses.

Welcome to the modern uses of Vinegar in 'Be Your Own Doctor With Apple Cider Vinegar'.

APPLE CIDER VINEGAR AND HER SISTERS.

Vinegar is produced from the fermentation of a variety of materials including wine, cereals such as barley, rice, and cider.

The first stage is to ferment the chosen material to alcohol which is later distilled to Vinegar.

The alcohol is ethanol while the acid produced is acetic acid, the main ingredient of vinegar besides water.

Apple Cider Vinegar is made from the fermentation of raw apple.

It will thus be clear that vinegar comes from sugar containing materials which are fermented into alcohol before oxygen is introduced to the system to convert it into vinegar.

If the first stage of fermentation is bypassed, whatever is produced cannot qualify to be called vinegar.

Initially, it took weeks or even months to produce vinegar but chemistry, technology and mechanization have combined together to speed up the process as you can now get vinegar made in a matter of days.

Vinegar is sour in taste. And the word vinegar was derived from the French word vinaigre, meaning "sour wine."

The main ingredient of vinegar is Acetic Acid (CH3COOH) or Ethanoic Acid, even though there may be traces of other acids such as malic, tartaric, and citric acids.

So, if we want to talk about the chemistry of vinegar, we will be discussing the

chemistry of Acetic Acid.

Acetic acid is a weak organic acid that differentiates it from inorganic acids such as sulphuric acid used for electrolytes and hydrochloric acid used for bleaching.

Carbonic acids are made from alcohol. For example, Acetic acid is made from ethanol by removing the OH group and replacing it with oxygen.

The more oxygen atoms in an organic acid the more powerful it becomes. Thus Acetic acid is more powerful than Formic acid. (HCOOH)

$$C_2H_5OH + O_2 \rightarrow CH_3COOH + H_2O$$

Generally, the acetic acid in Vinegar ranges from 4 to 8 percent in volume for general uses but when they are used for pickling, the percentage may go as high as 14 percent.

The pH of vinegar is usually between 2.5 and 3 depending on what it is meant for.

Density is 0.9gm/cm3 which makes it slightly lighter than water. Water has a density of 1.0gm/cm3

TYPES OF VINEGAR.

Apple Cider Vinegar.
This is the grandmother, the grandma of all kinds of vinegar which is also called cider vinegar because it is made from apple or apple cider.

Brownish in color and often sold unfiltered with Mother. It is capable of many uses.

Balsamic vinegar
Usually, for the upper-class citizens in Italy, Balsamic vinegar is made from white grapes which are slowly fermented.

It is aromatic, which means the acid group is attached to a benzene group.

This vinegar has a high concentration of acid but the aromatic properties mellow down the sourness.

Labour intensive in production but modern technology has sped up the process and it's now not limited to the upper class alone.

Malt vinegar

Malting barley is the main raw material to produce Malt vinegar. The starch in the grain is fermented to maltose which is then processed to vinegar and then aged.

The colour is light brown also with a sour taste like all kinds of vinegar.

Usually used as a condiment and if you ever feel a sour taste while eating Fish and Chips in the UK, you can be sure you are eating Malt vinegar.

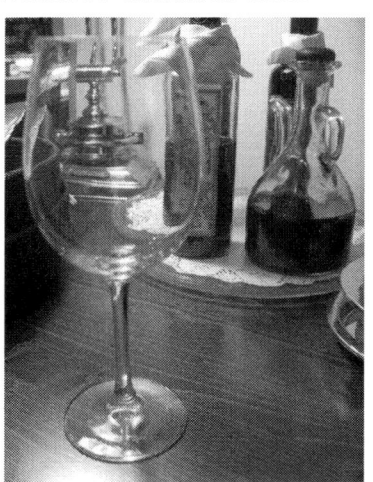

Rice vinegar

Rice vinegar is made from rice and is common with people in the East. It can be in various colors, white, light yellow, and red.

The Japanese use Rice vinegar for their sushi rice and also salad dressings

White vinegar.

White Vinegar is next in popularity to Apple Cider Vinegar. It is made from grains mainly, with Maize being the major.

The appearance is transparent.

After the fermentation, it is distilled under high heat, the droplets collected and allowed to cool down to make the white vinegar that is almost pure Acetic acid.

Used for culinary and household cleaning purposes because of its high acidity level.

Most white vinegar sold is about 5% volume acetic acid which is higher than that of Apple Cider Vinegar.

Wine vinegar,
Wine vinegar is made from wine, red or white, and is common in central Europe and Mediterranean countries.

They are less acidic than White vinegar and Apple Cider Vinegar.

The more mature they are, the more expensive.

The above are major kinds of vinegar, but there are lesser-known ones such as Cane Vinegar, coconut vinegar, fruit vinegar, flavored and Raisin and date vinegar,

In **'Be Your Own Doctor With Apple Cider Vinegar'**, readers to use raw Apple Cider Vinegar with the mother

DIFFERENCES BETWEEN APPLE CIDER VINEGAR AND WHITE VINEGAR.

Are Apple Cider Vinegar and white vinegar the same?

Yes, and No.

Yes, to the extent that they may be used interchangeably in some cases, and no, to the extent that they differ in appearance and source of preparation.

Apple Cider Vinegar is made from apple, while white vinegar is made from other materials such as a cereal but both have acetic acid as their main active ingredient, with minute quantity of citric acid.

Apple Cider Vinegar may also contain Malic acid and some amounts of carbohydrates. Apple Cider Vinegar is fat and protein-free.

For the record, there are many types of vinegar depending on the raw material used to make them. (See Types of Vinegar above)

Some other kinds of vinegar include cane vinegar from cane, malt vinegar from malt, wheat or barley, and coconut vinegar from coconut.

All kinds of vinegar are made through the chemical process of fermentation using alcohol or bacteria producing acetic acid.

For example, Apple Cider Vinegar is made from the fermentation of apple while coconut vinegar is made from the fermentation of coconut.

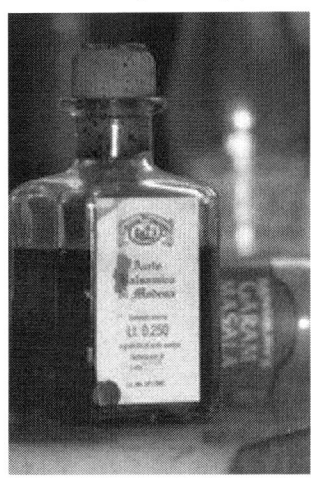

The process of fermentation can last for months depending on the final product in mind.

But in modern days, a catalyst called 'a mother' can be added to speed up the process which makes the production of vinegar possible in a matter of days.

A mother is a bacteria culture that adds oxygen to the process to speed it up.

Most Apple Cider Vinegar have a mother incorporated in them and could be seen at the bottom of the bottle.

The two commonest kinds of vinegar are white vinegar and Apple Cider Vinegar.

ACV is gentler, less acidic, and is the one used for medicinal purposes while white vinegar is more acidic and therefore more corrosive with lower pH and it is the one generally used for other uses outside medicine.

For medicinal uses, Apple Cider Vinegar is more potent.

In appearance, Apple Cider Vinegar is brownish in color while white vinegar is plain which gives you a simple way to identify them.

Let us recoup what we have been saying so far.

1. Both kinds of vinegar are made through the chemical process of fermentation of the raw material to alcohol, possibly ethanol, and the distillation of the ethanol to acetic acid, the main constituent of both kinds of vinegar with traces of some other weak acids like citric and malic acids.

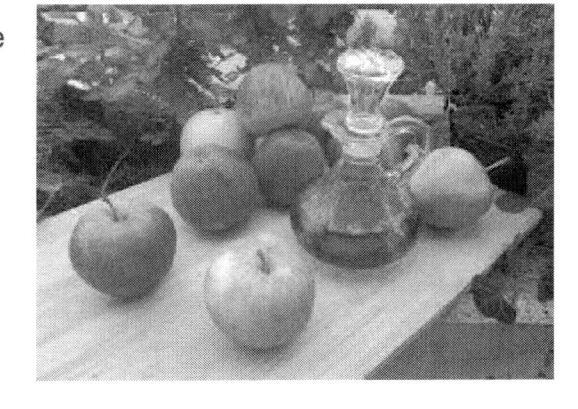

2. Most other kinds of vinegar are made from cereals like barley to get white vinegar while Apple Cider Vinegar is made only from apple cider.

3. As we said earlier, white vinegar tends to be mostly used as a cleaning agent while Apple Cider Vinegar is used for medicinal purposes.

White vinegar has a pH of about 2,5 or less which makes it more acidic than Apple Cider Vinegar with a pH of around 3.

This more acidic property of white vinegar lends it more to cleaning activities in the house and environment while the less acidic property of Apple Cider Vinegar pulls it toward health issues.

Most kinds of vinegar out there are white and do not have the ability to perform the health functions in this book.

Those white solutions in the bottles were so produced by manufacturers to please consumers as they do not like the look and the pungent smell of Apple Cider Vinegar.

Unfortunately, by removing these properties, manufacturers have stripped the vinegar of her health assisting properties.

Manufactures are happy and the undiscerning consumers are too. Consolation is that consumers can use these kinds of vinegar for non-health issues.

For the purpose of this book, read vinegar as (Apple Cider Vinegar). Wherever we mention vinegar be sure we are referring to (Apple Cider Vinegar).

DOCTORS, DO THEY ALWAYS TELL US THE WHOLE TRUTH?

Doctors deserve all the respect we give them.

Is it the long years of training or the special prerequisite of high cerebral acumen or the special qualities like extreme patience and accommodation they have to exhibit every minute they are on call?

They are a special breed but do they always tell us the whole truth?

Truth be told, there are some medical cases that are so clear even to the dumbest of laymen.

For example, a broken bone will need an orthopedic surgeon to set and restore it to normal.

To have a baby, you will need a doctor for a caesarean operation, if the bundle of joy refuses to come out of her cocoon.

A rotten foot as a result of diabetes will need the surgeon to amputate if the patient wants to live.

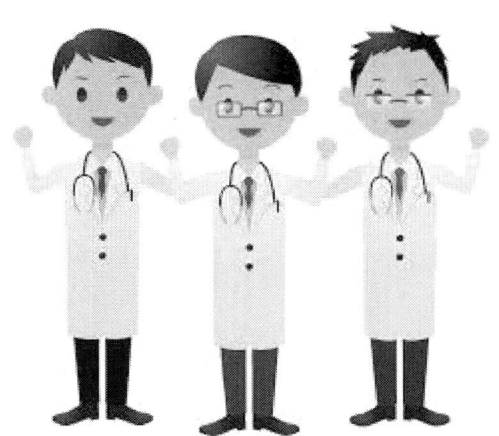

But unfortunately, there are some instances where and when we are not told the whole truth.

For instance, up till today, many people believe that the treatment which orthodox medicine has to offer for cancer patients will probably kill the patient before the cancer.

Many believe that chemotherapy, a common treatment for cancer which results in hair loss among other side effects is deadlier than cancer itself.

So also are the other cancer treatments such as Radiation therapy, Immunotherapy, Bone marrow transplant, and Hormone therapy.

What about diabetes? The story is similar, which is the cause of so many alternative medicine videos and adverts on the internet debunking orthodox medicine cure for diabetes.

Here is one of such advertisement, **'Diabetes, The Truth The Doctors Don't Want You To Know'**

The bottom line is that there are cheap alternatives to many expensive treatments recommended by our Doctors for many of these ailments.

And since they are there to make money while saving lives, they are not likely to tell us all the truth all the time.

When I asked a doctor friend why they have to prescribe medicines for all ailments when rest or a simple home remedy would have sufficed, his answer was very pragmatic probably because he was talking to a friend. 'We all go to the same market' he said. And that is the truth.

Save for accidents or emergencies, there are home remedies for many of the small ailments we go to the hospital for, but unfortunately, many of us are not aware.

When we know, some of us think they are too educated and sophisticated to believe in these things.

In many instances, the medics will tell you such treatments are not supported by scientific evidence. They have forgotten that alternative medicine predated orthodox medicine.

Fortunately, what medics think does not change the truth.

If Hydrogen Peroxide, suppresses whitlow as it does, all the medics in this world cannot change that.

They cannot change the truth that vinegar and ginger defeat constipation and indigestion probably better than the expensive drugs they prescribe.

The combo of Doctors and Pharmacists is one that has been licensed to eat-up the masses. You cannot blame them; it is expensive to produce either.

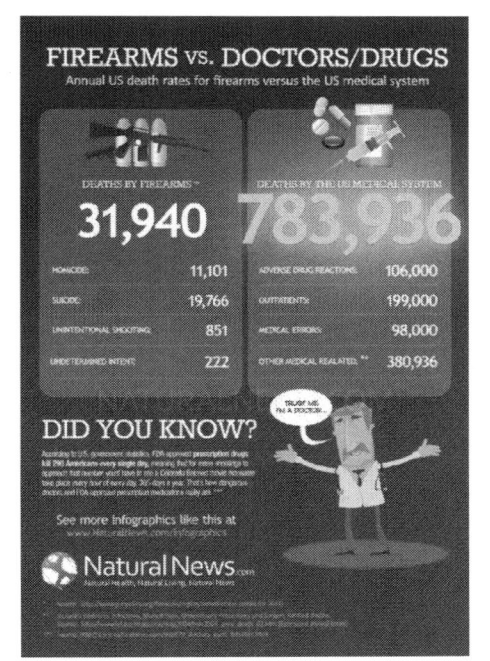

Let us have a look at some stats that may shock you as they did me.

Do you know that there are more deaths caused by doctors than firearms? You don't believe, I did not too till I read this:

Let us make a quick dash to naturalnews.com. It all started as a joke that doctors kill more than firearms carriers.

But in 2013, naturalnews.com's Mike Adams introduced figures into the debate in an article titled, "Doctors kill 2,450% more Americans than all gun-related deaths combined,"

He claimed that in a 2011 study, there were 783,936 deaths attributed to Doctors and 31,940 deaths by firearms out of which 19,766 were suicide meaning that only 12,174 were deliberate killings.

Now that means you are 64 times more likely to be killed by your doctor and drugs than by a bullet.

The Doctors and Pharmacists do not kill you by firing a rifle or deliberately injecting you with lethal substances, but they slowly kill you with treatments such as chemotherapy, vaccines and drugs, and errors.

This is quoted from the naturalnews.com info graph.

'According to USA government statistics, FDA approved drugs kill 290 Americans every single day, meaning that for mass shooting to approach that, you will have to see a Colorado batman movie massacre every hour every day, 365 days a year. That is how dangerous Doctors and FDA approved prescription medications really are-'

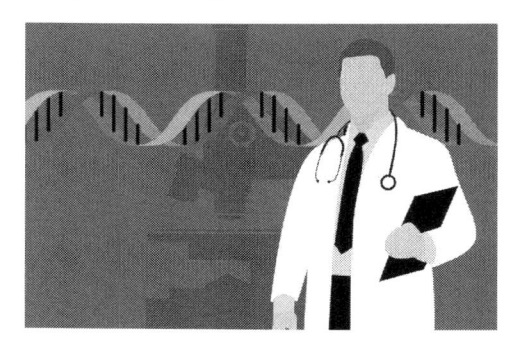

We should not get this wrong, doctors are our friends so are the Pharmacists, but they are humans and there could be human errors and don't forget 'we go to the same market'

Why do you think they talk about side effects in medicine?

Some drugs will cure a disease only to leave the patient with two or three other diseases which will ensure he visits the doctor regularly.

Many people believe that drugs used for cancer do affect the kidney and the lungs, two vital organs for the human body.

So, of what use is a cancer-free body with almost dead kidneys and lungs and probably the liver which is the most vital after the heart?

We are not saying these to make you hate the doctors.

No, they are our friends and sometimes we cannot do without them but there are a lot we can do for ourselves cheaply which reduces our visits to them greatly or eliminates it altogether.

This is why you have to be conversant with the simple medicinal uses of cheap substances like Vinegar, Baking Soda.

Many naturalists believe that if you were to choose two household items that have high practicability combined with usefulness, it would be Vinegar and Hydrogen Peroxide. I add Baking Soda to make three.

Undoubtedly, vinegar is believed to be one of nature's biggest gifts to mankind.

Welcome to the worlds of Vinegar. Go ahead and Be Your Own Doctor With Apple Cider Vinegar

SIX DON'TS WITH APPLE CIDER VINEGAR.

Contemporary and Alternative Medicine and Conventional Medicine are not the best of friends which is the reason they want to shoot CAM down.

No matter how hard they try, there are evidences daily that CAM has come to stay.

That is why practitioners and users have to thread softly so as not to arm orthodox medicine with the weapons to shoot CAM down.

Many proven uses of natural substances are always debunked with 'there are no scientific proofs' even when they know they work.

There may not be proofs, but that doesn't say they don't work.

For example, they say Hydrogen Peroxide does not dry up whitlow when there are many who could swear by it including me.

There may be a temptation to rush things because of anxiety, please don't.

Never do these six things with Apple Cider Vinegar

1. Never Drink ACV Straight.

It may not kill you if you take it straight, but may cause serious discomfort. Apple Cider Vinegar is acidic, so always dilute with water.

Drinking it undiluted may damage your teeth enamel and lining of the mouth and throat.

2. Little At A Time, At The Beginning.

When you are starting Apple Cider Vinegar therapy for the first time, go a little at a time and watch for allergies.

Our anatomies are not the same, so watch how your body reacts to the therapy. If there is no problem, then go ahead and follow the therapy fully.

3. On The Skin, Do A Patch Test First.

As in 2 above, do it little at a time. If for example, you want to apply ACV solution on your skin whether to tone the face or exfoliate the skin, test a small portion of your forearm before you apply on the face.

If you do not feel any burns or allergies go the full length.

If you do, discontinue or add more water and test again.

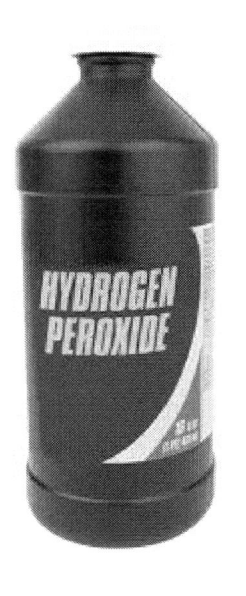

4. Don't Mix With Other Strong Chemicals.

Apple Cider Vinegar is strong and astringent enough to mix with other astringent materials such as Salicylic acid and others.

The result will be counterproductive. Mix only with substances gentle on the skin like lemon, aloe vera, etc.

5. Hydrogen Peroxide.

Don't ever; ever mix with Hydrogen peroxide under any circumstance. As a disinfectant, you may use one after the other but not together. Mixing them together produces Peracetic acid, a very corrosive substance.

6. Daily Ingestion.

Don't ingest more than 2 tablespoons a day.

THE USES OF ACV.

1. Acid Reflux: Very Discomforting.

Acid reflux, Heart Burn & Gastroesophageal Reflux Disease (GERD) are similar

The three are similar but they are not the same.

Let Us differentiate the three.

Acid Reflux is when the food in your stomach keeps moving up and down and at times to as high as the throat giving you some hot feeling in the thoracic cavity (the chest). This hot sensation in the chest is called heartburn.

You are likely going to have acid reflux if you have just eaten a heavy meal, or after a meal of spicy food, or eating while lying down.

These are some of the symptoms of Acid Reflux but may differ from person to person.

Heartburn as we said above.

Regurgitation.

Bloating.

A problem in swallowing.

Bitter taste.

When Acid Reflux and heartburn occur twice or more in a week, the situation is called GERD or

Gastroesophageal Reflux Disease. Symptoms include those mentioned above and difficulty in breathing and cough.

These are some of the causes of GERD

- Fatness

- Smoking
- Pregnancy
- Hernia.
- Heavy food and going to bed immediately after such a meal.
- Using pain killers like Ibuprofen And Aspirin
- Consumption of alcohol, soda, or coffee

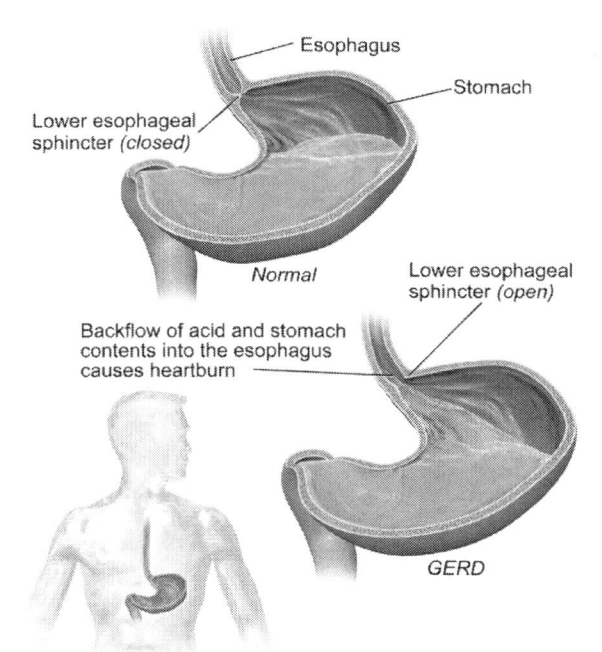

Gastroesophageal Reflux Disease (GERD)

Theory Of Vinegar Cure For Acid Reflux

Some people do not understand how you can use vinegar which contains acid to fight Acid Reflux.

They may be right, but with some explanations, they will realize why this is possible.

Remember also that Vinegar is antibacterial and it also consists of enzymes, pectin, and protein.

It is believed that vinegar will balance the acidity in the stomach and deal with acid reflux causing bacteria.

The enzymes and protein also help in fighting acid reflux.

Vinegar is such a complex compound consisting of many ingredients that will help in this fight against Acid Reflux.

How Do You Deal With Acid Reflux With Vinegar?

You will not be wrong if you try to use vinegar to treat your heartburn and acid reflux. You will get with it many additional gains as you will discover in this book.

Vinegar is useful to fight excess weight and high blood pressure and many other medicinal issues. It is a gain-gain situation.

The liquid apple vinegar works but the pills work as well. For your acid reflux treatment, we recommend the pills with your meal.

The pills have amino acids and antioxidants just like the liquid Apple Cider Vinegar to give you the same health benefits.

For ACV use, just sip some diluted solution of Apple Cider Vinegar and water now and then.

Removing tight clothes, standing straight, and elevating your trunk will help to ease Acid Reflux.

If you still have these feelings after 2 weeks, you will need to see your doctor, that is the cliché but more often than not you will not need to.

2. Acne Astringent: Not Ok For Your Face.

Acnes are blemishes that appear on the face, neck, back, and chest or anywhere on the upper side of the body.

Sufferers look for solutions that are available in form of creams, liquids or soaps, and other over-the-counter products.

The problem is that they may be made of toxic chemicals which may cause other issues besides being expensive.

Apple Cider Vinegar can give you tremendous help here and could be used in form of a tub bath, facial mask, tonic, or topical application.

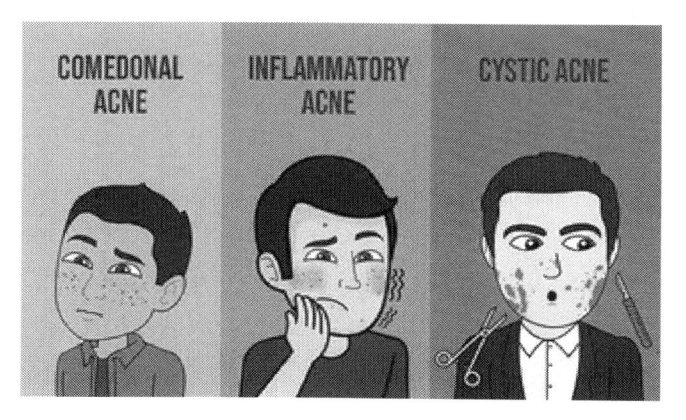

Elsewhere, we talked about skin toning in this book. You can use the same principle to fight off Acne.

Apple Cider Vinegar will fight the bacteria and other organisms causing problems on the skin.

ACV effect is more noticeable on oily skins because as an astringent, it will remove excess oil in addition to opening blocked pores.

Apply Apple Cider Vinegar diluted with water (50/50 ratio) on the spots with cotton wool or hand towel and see them disappear. Leave on the skin for some minutes.

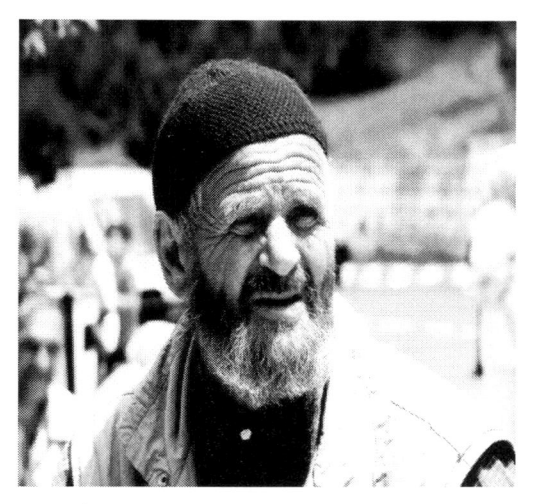

This applies to acne, pimples, and even scars which get removed to bring back your confidence.

Alternatively, add three cups of Apple Cider Vinegar to the tub full of water and soak there for about thirty minutes.

You may leave diluted vinegar on your face overnight for the best result.

3.Age Spots And Wrinkles: Remove Them.

As we grow old, having age spots and wrinkles is inevitable. Apple Cider Vinegar helps us to remove these spots and those fine lines called wrinkles.

Lightening the dark spots should not surprise us because vinegar is acidic and acids will lighten pigmentation.

Apply a mixture of an equal volume of ACV and water on the spots, leave on for about 10 minutes or longer, wash off, and dry up. You may repeat if the spots are stubborn.

Why would you go for cryosurgery when Apple Cider Vinegar can help.

4.Ageing: Reverse Your Age.

Precipitated acid crystals cause cramps and premature aging.

We must all fight its build up in the body and its greatest antidote is flushing.

ACV, honey and distilled water conquer acid crystals build up.

Make a cocktail from the three (Apple Cider Vinegar, Honey, and distilled water) drink three to five times daily.

Add to this about 5 glasses of distilled water in a day.

The toxins will be flushed out through the excretory organs in the body.

4. Allergies: Stop Them.

Allergies are most commonly caused by irritants or reactions to some stimulants not in tandem with the system.

They could show up as itchy eyes, running nose, burning throat, mucus production, and more.

Because they are often mild, sufferers result to over-the-counter products which give temporary relief with the symptoms returning later.

These products cost money besides the possibility of side effects.

Apple Cider Vinegar fights allergies using its antiviral, antibacterial, and antiseptic abilities.

Adding it to your diet reduces the production of mucus and cures sinus.

These are signs of a distressed immune system. Apple Cider Vinegar assists in reducing the build-up of these.

Alternatively, you can make a drink of one tablespoon of Apple Cider Vinegar, one teaspoon of honey, one teaspoon of cinnamon in a cup of hot water and drink thrice daily.

If these symptoms are not fought early, they could lead to serious illnesses such as sinus.

To prevent this, you may need a preventive dose of the above drink which is a cup of the above once a day.

5. Amino Acids: You Need Them.

Amino acids are the building blocks of protein taking part in the metabolic processes in the body.

They are in all the body cells with functions ranging from communication from the brain to other parts of the body to aiding digestion.

There are about 10 essential amino acids that we cannot manufacture as differentiated from the non-essential amino acids.

The essential amino acids are the ones we need in the body.

The body does not store amino acids as it does foods like fats and carbohydrates which makes it compulsory for us to take it every day.

You do not have to ingest amino acids directly to have essential amino acids in your system as you can get them from other sources.

You will get enough amount of amino acid by eating animal-based foods such as milk, meat, eggs, and fish.

There are also plant-based foods such as soybeans, Spirulina (Plant Algae) Spinach, New Zealand Spinach, and nuts such as Pumpkin Seeds providing amino acids.

Diets spiced with Apple Cider Vinegar will make the body absorb amino acids rapidly, besides the fact that it has some amino acids itself.

Recipe.

Two teaspoons Apple Cider Vinegar,
One teaspoon of honey,
One cup of water.

Drink thrice daily for your body to maximize its amino acid intake and utilization.

6. Antibacterial Properties: Bacteria In Serious Trouble.

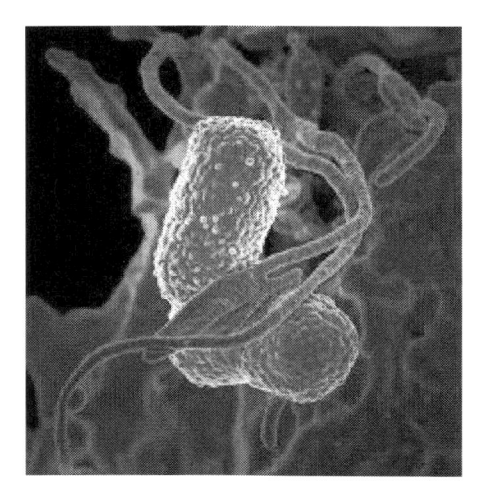

Acetic acid being the major constituent of Apple Cider Vinegar not only has antibacterial properties, but it also kills Staphylococcus Aureus and Escherichia Coli, two bacteria causing infection in the urinary tract.

It was also found out that Apple Cider Vinegar Kills Enterococcus Faecal is, a bacterium in human guts and bowels which cause infection.

Refer to Detoxification and Immunity.

7. Antifungal Properties: Kill The Fungi.

A mouth infection can be life-threatening especially with type 2 diabetes patients who are derelict in controlling their sugar levels.

Common fungal infections in humans are found in the throat and the virginal and are called Candida Albicans.

They can last very long and develop resistance to antifungal compounds.

Apple Cider Vinegar will assist.

In a study, a woman with serious 5 years' virginal candida got better with ACV.

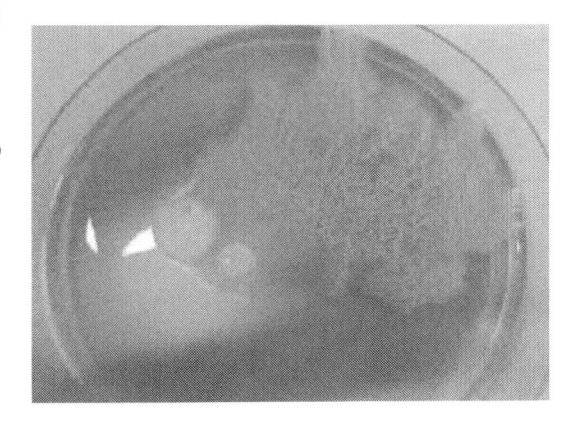

In another study, a man with type 2 diabetes with persistent mouth Candida applied Apple Cider Vinegar to the mouth twice a day for seven days.

At the end of the week, there was about a 94% reduction in the candida count.

By using ACV, people who wear dentures do get some relief from a candida species that cause denture stomatitis which is peculiar to them.

Apple Cider Vinegar kills them outright.

Gargle a solution of one teaspoon ACV in 250 mills of warm water and spit out.

Do not forget the daily drinking of the detox.

8. Appetite: Eat Less, Less Fatty.

Apple Cider Vinegar is known to suppress appetite and gives you some fullness if you ingest it. It promotes fullness and reduces the intake of calories.

Some people believe it's the enzymes in vinegar responsible for this function.

Others believe it's the Acetic Acid that slows the rate at which sugars are released to the bloodstream which makes you full.

Yet others say the pectin present in Apple Cider Vinegar is responsible.

One theory is that the acetic acid in Apple Cider Vinegar reduces the glycemic index of foods, which slows the appetite.

We may not know how it works, but we know it works.

This is a simple recipe.

One tablespoon ACV plus two cups of water. Whirl properly and sip for the whole day.

9. Artery Plaque Can Kill: Clear The Road For Blood.

When plaque made of cholesterol, fat, calcium, and others, is built in arteries, a disease called Atherosclerosis results.

With time, the plaque hardens and blocks the arteries making it narrower which limits the flow of blood rich in oxygen to the organs and the body.

Happily enough, we can unclog the artery using Apple Cider Vinegar and some other naturals such as ginger, lemon, etc.

- Lemon juice-Half Cup

- Apple cider vinegar-Half cup

- Garlic puree –Half a cup

- Organic Honey-One cup.

- Ginger juice –Half a cup

Extract the juice, using medium heat, heat them together without the honey for about thirty minutes. Cool off completely, then add the honey and mix properly.

Put in the fridge and drink one spoon at a time on an empty stomach thrice a day.

Free blood flow for you.

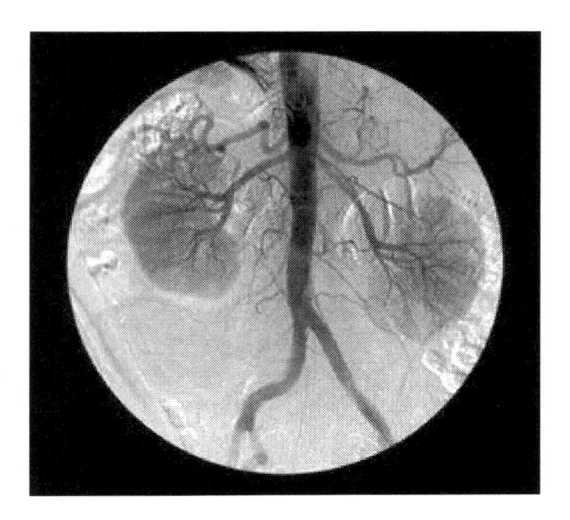

10. Asthma: Get Clear Airways.

Sufferers of Asthma or COPD (Chronic Obstructive Pulmonary Disease) can get help with Apple Cider Vinegar.

Using Apple Cider Vinegar builds immunity and enhances respiratory functions. With increased immunity, those suffering from Asthma will be able to fight the symptoms.

The steam and applied treatments are known to be effective in reducing the severity of asthmatic symptoms.

Steam Treatment.

Get one cup Apple Cider Vinegar and Four cups water. Boil in a pot.

Bring down the pot and put your face over the hot solution not forgetting to cover your head and the pot with a big towel and inhale the steam coming out and see your airways cleared.

Drink:

One cup of water.
One tablespoon Apple Cider Vinegar.
Half cup freshly juiced ginger
Mix and drink once a day.

11. Athletes Foot: Wipe It Off.

Athletes' foot is a fungal infection, a sort of ringworm between the toes and on the sole.

Whitish or pinkish colour accompanied with itches.

If you have this infection, you can trust Apple Cider Vinegar to help. Make a vinegar bath with Apple Cider Vinegar from an equal volume of water and ACV and soak the feet there or you make a more concentrated one and apply directly. Soak for 15minutes and repeat twice daily depending on its intensity.

Please, remember not to use vinegar directly. You can mix a tablespoon with sixty-five tablespoons of water and apply directly.

Use ACV with the mother for a permanent result.

You may need to wash your socks with water and some quantity of Apple Cider Vinegar to prevent a recurrence.

Let me give you this for free. Get some powder of Baking soda also called Sodium Bicarbonate, make a paste with it, and apply directly. Sure to defeat athlete's foot.

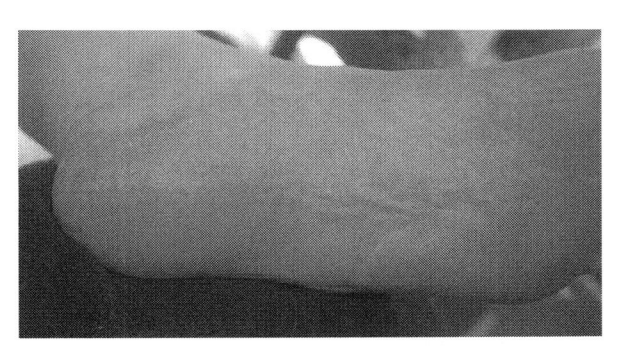

13.Backache: Straighten Up.

Backache gives you a problem which affects the whole body. Whether you are sitting, walking, or standing, it gives pain that reduces your productivity.

Backache is caused by inflammation of the tissues, muscles, bones, and nerves. And as we know that, Apple Cider Vinegar fights inflammation, it is natural to expect it to give you relief from your backache

Remember that ACV contains potassium, magnesium, calcium, and phosphorous which help to reduce bone pain as these minerals are essential in bone toughness.

If you want to do the tub bath, get your tab full with water, and add three cups of Apple Cider Vinegarr. Soak yourself in the tab for thirty minutes.

Alternatively, if you prefer the drink put one tablespoon of ACV in a cup of water and drink once a day.

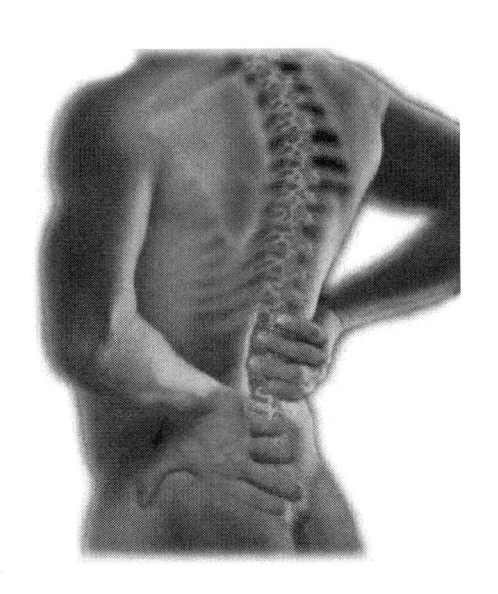

14. Bacterial Cystitis: Clear The Tract.

Bacteria Cystitis is another term for Urinary Tract Infection (UTI) which gives sufferers some tingling sensation.

It makes sufferers feeling to urinate frequently with or without urine coming out, giving a burning sensation along the tract.

This condition is commonly caused by bacteria and is usually treated with antibiotics.

However, you also have Interstitial Cystitis which is caused by inflammation of the wall of the bladder giving the same symptoms as Bacteria Cystitis

But why going for expensive antibiotics with their possible side effects when your natural Apple Cider Vinegar is there to cure the Bacteria Cystitis?

Prepare one teaspoon of Apple Cider Vinegar in about 240mils of water. Drink piecemeal about 6 times a day to make you urinate to flush out harmful bacteria.

You can also add about 2 tablespoons to the food of your medium-sized dog. However, do this sparingly.

15. Bedwetting: Too Bad, Stop It.

If you bed wet once in a while, there may not be anything to worry about as anxiety or deep sleep may cause it.

However, if it is persistent, the condition is called Nocturnal Enuresis and may be caused by UTI or bladder infection.

If you urinate too much, it means your Bladder is making more urine than necessary.

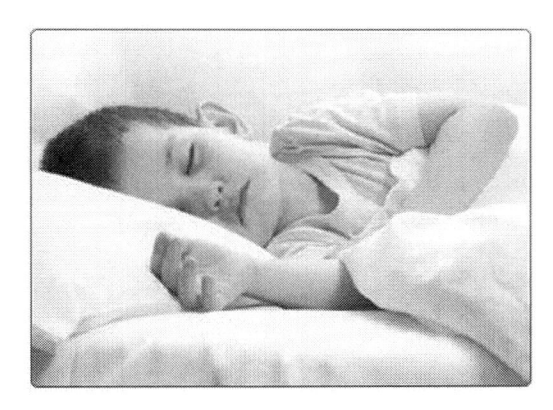

Another cause of too much urine is a type of diabetes called Diabetes Insipidus.

If you drink too much beer before going to bed, you will definitely pee many times and may bed wet when you sleep deeply.

Obviously, the first precaution against bedwetting is to run away from anything liquid at least three hours before sleeping.

Mix two teaspoons of Apple Cider Vinegar with one teaspoon of honey before bed. Also, imprint it on your mind you will not bed wet.

You will soon find out you do not bed wet again.

This can also be used for kids bedwetting

16. Bites: Soothe The Pains.

There are many home remedies for insect bites and I am happy to announce that vinegar is there with them.

To be sure, you can use Baking Soda salt, Lemon, Aloe Vera, and even cold water to reduce the itches and inflation but Apple Cider Vinegar does it best.

ACV with its aid and enzymes soothes the pain and its sharp smell and taste keep insects away from you.

So if you are stung by a spider or an insect, just apply some drops of diluted vinegar on the spot.

The sting will go and inflammation will reduce.

If it is severe, you may soak a small towel with vinegar solution and cover the place for some time.

If you cannot lay your hands on Apple Cider Vinegar with the mother quickly, white vinegar will do.

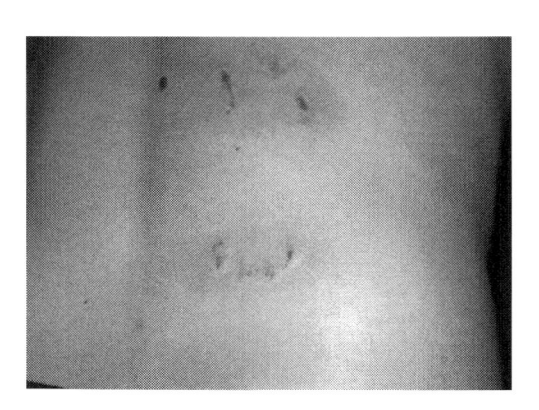

17. Bleeding: Stop The Flow.

There are available studies showing that an Apple Cider Vinegar soaked bandages stop bleeding and prevent infection

18. Blood Sugar: High Sugar, Big Problem.

You can use Apple Cider Vinegar to control your blood sugar level.

Too much sugar in one's blood, one of which is Type 2 diabetes will lead to heart problems.

People with such medical conditions may have problems with body organs such as the eye, kidney, nervous system, sex urge and chest.

To stem this, sufferers have to reduce their sugar level in the blood and experiments have shown that Apple Cider Vinegar can help.

Some small sample studies of people consuming ACV for about 10 weeks show a reduction in their sugar level.

Another showed that those who eat meals with Apple Cider Vinegar showed a reduction in triglyceride and insulin after the meal more than those who did not eat with ACV.

There is no agreed recipe for using Apple Cider Vinegar but it is agreed that you do not ingest it undiluted.

In the dietary treatment of Sugar reduction, food with fibers is recommended and Apple Cider Vinegar has its own dose of fiber with other substances such as enzymes, minerals, and nutrients which help in detoxifying the body.

In this case, one teaspoon of Apple Cider Vinegar in 250 mills of water will do. If the taste is too sour, you are free to add some quantity of honey.

Mix thoroughly and drink three times daily.

19. Bronchitis: Clear The Mucus.

If you are looking for a great enemy of throat germs and mucus, do not look further than Apple Cider Vinegar.

Gargle a solution of a glass of water and one teaspoon of ACV once in three hours and spit out as you do want to swallow the germs and toxins.

Add to this hot Apple Cider Vinegar press on the throat by using an ACV soaked towel and use a hot water bottle to heat the area.

Apple Cider Vinegar gargle twice a week is good even when you are in good health.

I do this often to clear the way.

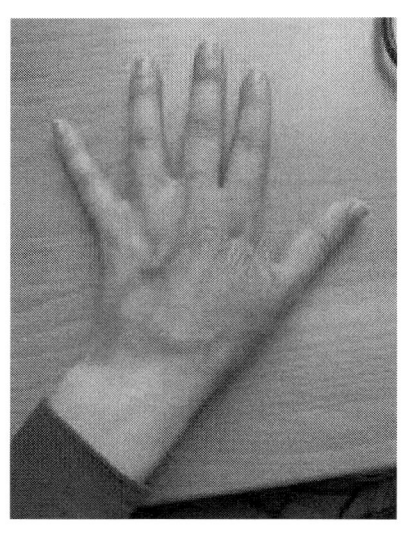

20. Burns: Any Type Of Burns.

You are surprised that acidic Apple Cider Vinegar will heal burns instead of aggravating it? You are forgiven as many think similarly.

But on the contrary, ACV is a complex substance. It contains enzymes, minerals, and other constituents that not only give relieve from burns but also prevent infection.

Mix equal volume of water and ACV and apply with cotton wool on the blisters and they will dry out.

One of the users of raw Apple Cider Vinegar who always have a bottle not only in the kitchen but also in the car says splashing ACV on raw burns give instant soothing, stops the pain completely, reduces inflammation before beginning the healing process, also preventing infection and scarring

Burns could be hot water splash, heater burn, or even car engine and exhaust burn.

Make a mixture of Half a cup of Apple Cider Vinegar, two cups of water. Dab the affected area with the solution for about fifteen minutes and repeat about 4 times within three hours.

You can also wrap the area loosely with a bandage or gauze soaked with the ACV solution made as above.

Bonus. A 50/50 mixture of Baking Soda and water will also give a quick soothing effect. Or just sprinkle Baking Soda powder on the burn.

You now see why you should have a bottle of raw Apple Cider Vinegar in your kitchen and your car. If I were you I will add dirt-cheap Baking Soda as well.

21. Calcium and Potassium Absorption: So, So Important.

It is agreed that strong bones need Calcium and Potassium.

But does Apple Cider Vinegar aid the absorption of these minerals? Let us consider what we know.

We know that ACV contains Acetic acid and some other mild acids.

These acids are considered to be strong enough to dissolve Calcium and Potassium which may render the bone soft and weak.

However, small doses of Apple Cider Vinegar as we said elsewhere here aid absorption of minerals meaning a small quantity of ACV may help in the absorption of these minerals to help the bones.

Osteoporosis, a disease meaning porous bone may be mitigated by using a small quantity of Apple Cider Vinegar in salad and other food dressings by exploiting its trophic effect which prevents bone turnover.

One Tablespoon ACV.
One Cup of Milk,
Half a cup of ice,
One Banana.

Mix in a blender and drink twice a week.

22. Cancer: Not Your Friend.

We will be brief about this. Cancer is a complex medical situation that cannot be fought off with a single therapy.

Even orthodox medicine fights it from many angles.

Some people can swear that Apple Cider Vinegar kills cancer cells but we won't here.

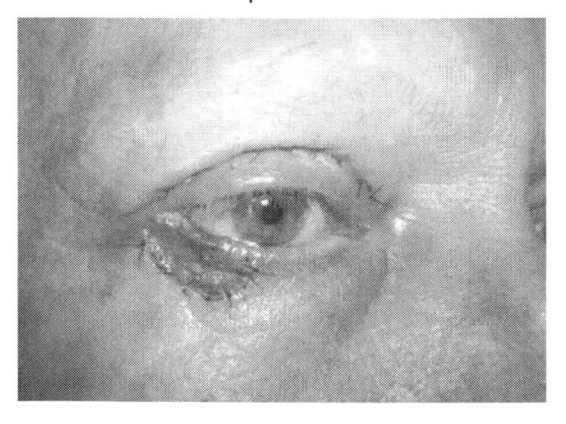

They believe, because of its acidic property which will help clean the esophagus thereby preventing oesophageal cancer, but this has not been proven.

Remember it is also claimed that Baking soda does fight cancer. It is neither here nor there.

However, using Apple Cider Vinegar as an additive to diets can prevent cancer cells from gathering together which is how far we can recommend.

Vitamin C, which is present in Apple Cider Vinegar may not cure cancer but may help in preventing it. It acts as an antioxidant, it increases immunity. These combine to reduce cancer infection.

You can make an Apple Cider Vinegar; vitamin C drink as follows.

One tablespoon Apple Cider Vinegar,

Half cup fresh grapefruit juice

One cup fresh orange juice

One cold banana

Blend in a blender and drink once a day.

Cancer-fighting photochemical are abundant in onions, beans, garlic, soybeans, legumes, cabbage, broccoli, cauliflower citrus fruits, etc. with tomatoes taking the trophy.

It may interest to note that, it is known that ingesting vinegar, not Apple Cider Vinegar gives some protective actions against cancer.

Consuming it may help to prevent cancer in the body system.

23. Cataracts: You Need Good Sight.

The eyes lighten up the body. Without the eyes, one is in perpetual darkness which makes it imperative to protect the eyes.

A cataract is a common disease of the eye and this is caused when the proteins in the eyes break down and hardened up to cover the eyes.

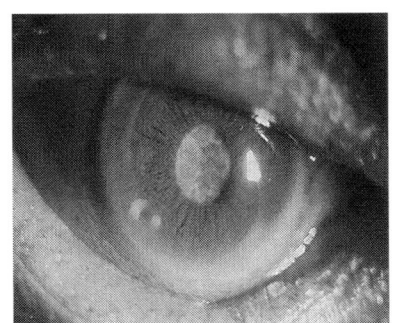

You see, the lens being the iris collects the light to the eyes. Long oxidative activities of the light, break down these substances which later harden up.

To prevent this means you have to include antioxidants in your meal over time.

So, you may not be able to use Apple Cider Vinegar to remove Cataracts, but you may use it to reduce your chances of having it by using Apple Cider Vinegar because it has antioxidants.

This recipe contains a substantial amount of antioxidant

One tablespoon Apple Cider Vinegar.

One cup of fresh carrot juice.

A quarter cup juice of ginger.

Blend and drink once a day

A family vast in healthy living and alternative therapy gives the following as a therapy for Cataract.

Three teaspoons of Apple Cider Vinegar to 250 mils of water. Use as eyewash or drops. Close the eye for about a minute.

For a start, you may use one teaspoon of ACV to 250 mills of water. Such high dilution will reduce the astringency of ACV.

24. Cellulite: Ugly Fats.

Those fats on the thighs and legs causing dimpling of the skin may be uncomfortable. They are called cellulite and Apple Cider Vinegar can take care of them.

Apply a mixture of one-part ACV and 2 parts water on cellulite regularly on the affected area and watch it disappear giving you a smooth thigh and legs you will be proud of.

You may add some honey to the mixture before rubbing in. Wash with water after about thirty minutes.

25. Cervical Cancer: Do A Dirt Cheap Test.

Cervical cancer is one of the commonest causes of death among women especially in the less developed parts of the world.

Yet there is a simple way to detect and cure it.

The pap-smear test for cervical cancer is the most common in the developed world, but it is expensive and could only be carried out by a medical doctor.

Alternatively, the Apple Cider Vinegar test is cheap and could be done by a nurse or even midwives.

The process is called visual inspection with Acetic Acid (VIA) and costs less than a dollar.

The cervix is swabbed with cotton wool soaked with vinegar (remember vinegar contains Acetic acid) which makes pre-cancerous spots turn white immediately.

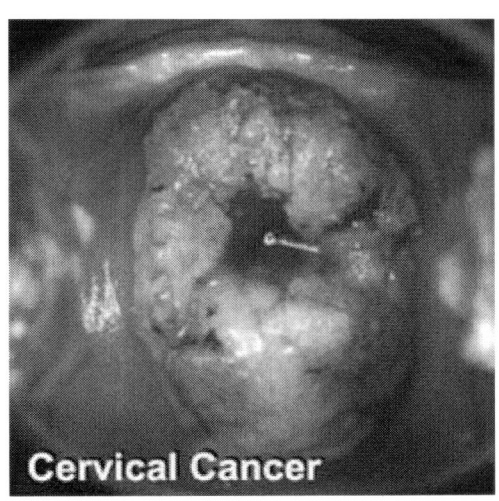

The spots can quickly be frozen up using a metallic probe cooled with dry ice, a process referred to as cryotherapy.

Cervical Cancer

26. Chickenpox : An Enemy of The Skin.

Chickenpox is usually the forerunner of Shingles and is caused by a virus called Herpes Zoster.

If you have had chickenpox, chances are that the virus is in you and should be treated.

They appear as very painful rashes and could be anywhere on the body and when severe, you may find it problematic to put on a shirt.

A dally drink of a tablespoon of Apple Cider Vinegar and a cup of water will prevent it.

If you have contacted it, deal with it with diluted ACV or a warm bath with it.

Fill the tub with water plus 3 cups of Apple Cider Vinegar.

Another Drink
One tablespoon ACV.
Half cup strawberries
One cup of green tea
Blend thoroughly and drink thrice a day.
See Shingles.

27. Cholesterol and Triglycerides: Cut Them Down.

Cholesterol level can be brought down with Apple Cider Vinegar.

We all know that too high cholesterol and triglyceride will eventually bring health issues.

These two substances at a high level increase the risk of heart attack and even stroke.

Happily enough, some studies carried out show that ACV consumption reduces the level of these two compounds.

Over a 12 weeks study, it was found out that those who took ACV with their meals showed weight loss in comparison to those who did not.

In addition, Apple Cider Vinegar users also had a reduction in the level of cholesterol and triglyceride.

Also, they (ACV users) showed a significant rise in their (HDL) High-Density Lipoprotein Cholesterol which doctors call good-cholesterol as it helps to reduce the risk of heart issues.

Apple Cider Vinegar has vitamins A, B, and C, plus magnesium, potassium, and a number of enzymes that help to maintain good health.

It also has a compound called pectin which attaches itself to cholesterol and moves it out of the body.

This drink fights cholesterol.

1 cup of water.
1 teaspoon Apple Cider Vinegar.

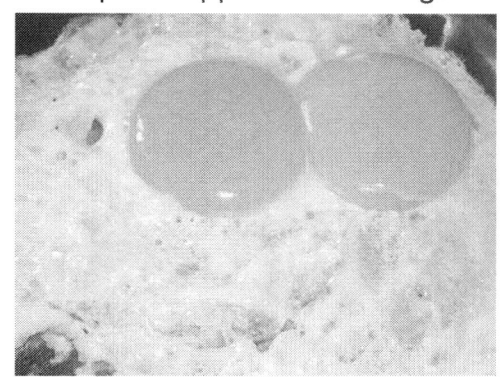

Drink two times daily.

Refer to usage under blood sugar reduction.

28. Conjunctivitis or Pink Eye: Get White Eyeballs.

Infection and/or inflammation of conjunctiva is referred to as conjunctivitis which appears as pink eyeballs.

Conjunctiva is the transparent membrane that covers the white section of the eye.

Keeping the eye moist is one of the functions of the conjunctiva.

Conjunctivitis is caused by bacterial and/or viral infection, but sometimes it could be as a result of eyes response to an allergy.

Symptoms include itching, eye redness, tearing, and watery discharge.

Conjunctivitis could be very contagious.

Treatment

If you have pink eye, Apple Cider Vinegar can help.

Use a very dilute solution. Say 10/90 of ACV and water as eye drops.

Apple Cider Vinegar is astringent, but when highly diluted like this, It does no harm to the eye while still doing its work.

See cataract.

29. Cough: Clear It Off.

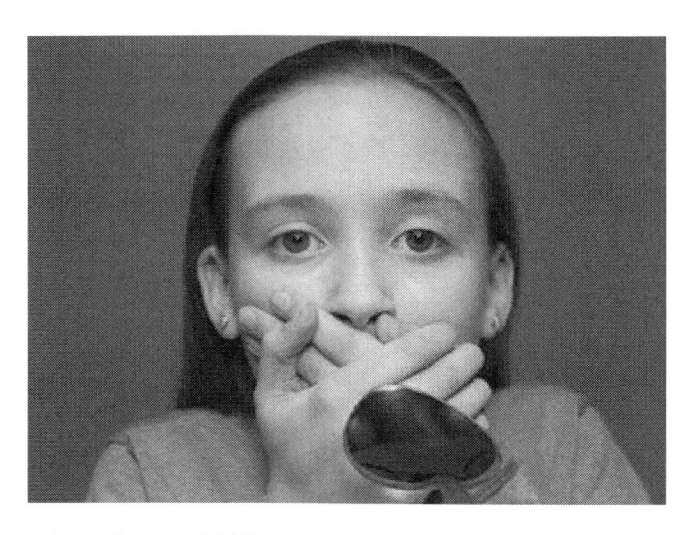

Dextromethorphan is an OTC drug for cough, and Mayo clinic says pure Honey is as effective.

Mix one tablespoon of pure raw honey with two tablespoons of top-quality Apple Cider Vinegar.

Drink twice a day to drive cough away.

30. Constipation: Too much Food, Too Much Junk.

Constipation is one of your greatest enemies.

Constipation produces toxins which are thrown back to the system by your liver because it cannot process it.

This goes on to cause diseases such as cancer, sickness, premature ageing, and lack of energy.

Living a healthy lifestyle can reduce the risk of constipation.

Stop eating processed and embalmed food, eat more fruits instead.

Apple Cider Vinegar contains pectin, malic acid, and of course Acetic acid.

Pectin is a fiber that is water-soluble which acts as a laxative.

Malic Acid and Acetic Acid are also digestion-friendly.

Therefore, ACV will help in relieving constipation.

Sip 50/50 solution of Apple Cider Vinegar and water.

To guide against constipation, drink plenty of water, eat more fibrous fruits, vegetables and nuts and abstain from caffeinated foods

31. Corns & Calluses: Ugly On Your Toes.

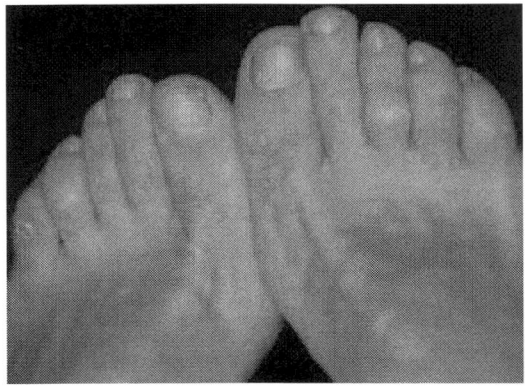

Corns & Calluses are raised skins caused by dead cells which occur as a result of persistent rubbing of the skin against a rough object.

It is common with toes of the feet when they have suffered consistent rubbing against the leather or covering of shoes.

Some people use pumice stones to clear this off, but you also have the option of Apple Cider Vinegar to soften the skin for removal and then regeneration of the skin.

Soak the feet in

Four liters of warm water
One cup ACV.
Thirty minutes, four times a day.

Scrape off.

32. Cradle Cap Cure: Give The Little One a Smooth Head.

Cradle cap on the head of babies does occur sometimes no matter how hard you try.

Do not worry, Apple Cider Vinegar will help you to remove it and you have a whistle clean head for your baby.

Mix water and ACV in a ratio of two to one. Apply on the baby's scalp for about 15 minutes and wash off later.

Do this twice a week until it goes.

Test a small portion of the head first and see if the bay reacts to this solution.

Please protect your baby's eyes.

33. Dandruff: Clear Off Ugly White Flakes.

Bottle Bacillus is the germ responsible for dryness of scalp and hair causing hair problems such as dandruff.

Each hair follicle has its own oil can which this germ clog into forming small dry crusts and dryness resulting in dandruff and itching.

You now have bristle hair which may now be falling off.

Apple Cider Vinegar in addition to killing the Bottle bacillus, also oils the hair bottles making the hairs lusher and more shine.

Mix equal parts of ACV and water to spray your scalp twice a week.

After spraying, wrap your towel around the hair for about an hour to allow the vinegar to do its work.

Hair properly wrapped, you could be doing other house chores.

One hour after, wash your hair normally.

Or

Put three tablespoons of Apple Cider Vinegar in 250mills of water, mix thoroughly, and part the hair to apply the solution directly to your scalp, and wrap your head using a towel.

34. Denture: Happy for A Good Soak.

Refrain from substances that are harsh on your denture and this includes Hydrogen Peroxide, bleach, white vinegar, and even some kinds of toothpaste.

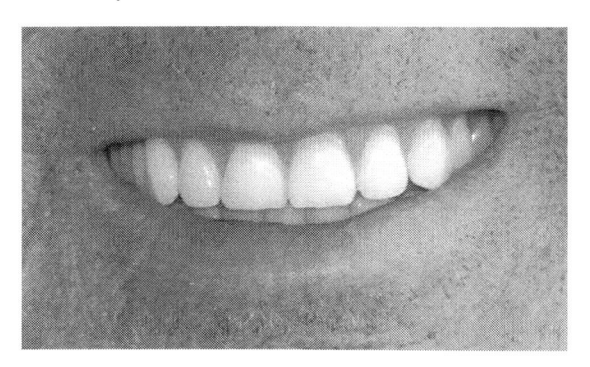

But you can use well-diluted Apple Cider Vinegar and even well diluted Baking soda to reduce their brashness.

Soak your dentures in the diluted solution for about thirty minutes to an hour or even overnight not forgetting to rinse thoroughly before re-inserting. They will thank you for this.

See Teeth.

35. Deodorant: Why Not Make Your Own.

A foul odor may be caused by sweating and bacteria especially in body areas not covered with cloth and where the air is restricted.

An example of such a place is the armpit.

Yes, there are proprietary products, but because of the after effect when these are absorbed into the system through the thin layer of the skin in the armpit, some users prefer the natural way.

A sure natural alternative is Apple Cider Vinegar,

ACV is sour and maybe smelly, but when it dries under your armpit, you get a pleasant odor.

It kills the bacteria oozing out the foul smell without the toxicity you get from using those proprietary products.

Apply a mixture of one tablespoon of Apple Cider Vinegar and one tablespoon of water to your armpit using cotton and allow to dry.

Alternatively, you could put this in a spraying bottle and spray directly.

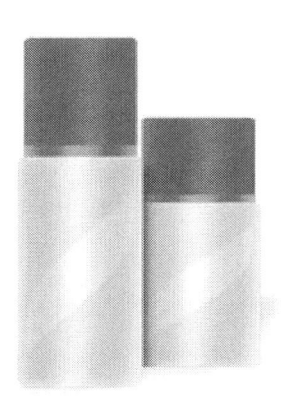

36. Detoxification: Get The Toxins Out.

Detoxification simply means removing toxins from the system and an Apple Cider Vinegar detoxification drink can help. These are some of the benefits you get when you detoxify.

- ➢ Your body is free of toxins you get from the environment, food, pollutants, etc.
- ➢ Assist body organs to get rid of wastes that had built up.

- ➢ Gives back to the body valuable minerals such as Potassium and vitamins for optimal performance.
- ➢ You get your share of Enzymes
- ➢ Spikes your immunity
- ➢ pH balance
- ➢ Weight control
- ➢ Smooth and healthy skin

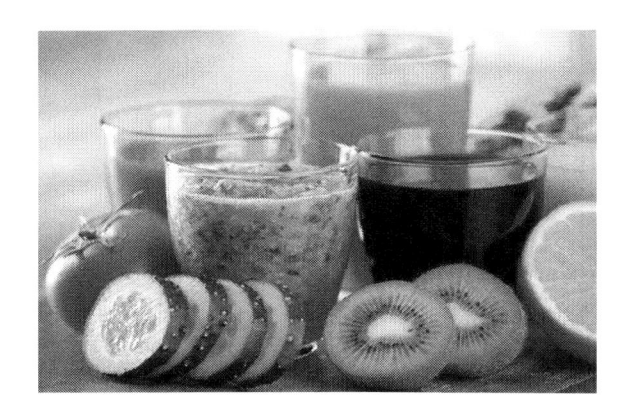

Apple Cider Vinegar Drink

- One Tablespoons apple cider vinegar

- Fresh lime Juice-One tablespoon

- Stevia-one teaspoon

- Water-2cups of cold water

Mix together thoroughly and drink.

Or

1. Two tablespoons of organic Apple Cider Vinegar.

2. One and half tablespoons of any sweetener such as maple syrup or honey

250mills of distilled water

Mix properly and drink.

Do this regularly and you will be free of these small ailments.

37. Diabetes: Balance Your Sugar Level.

It is agreed that too much insulin and glucose in the blood can lead to complications such as heart problems.

It is also agreed that Vinegar can help reduce the spike of these compounds in the bloodstream.

This is much better than different eating regimes recommended by million 'diabetes experts' on the net, which are most times very complicated and which may not give the desired results.

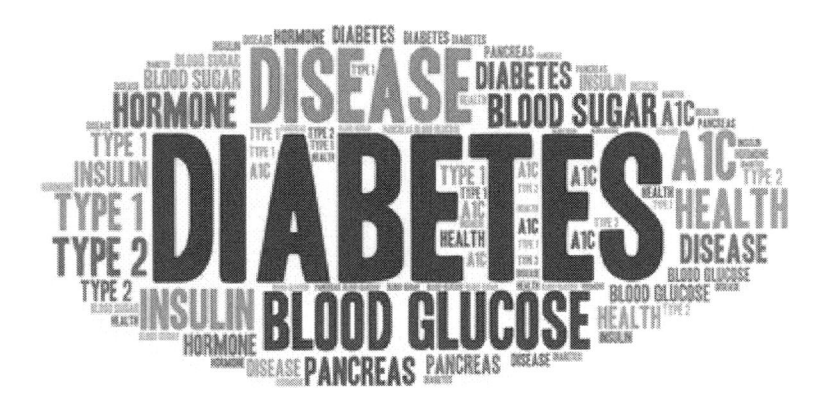

ACV with its enzymes and other constituents help Diabetic patients to balance their food intake to reduce the sugar level.

In a study by Prof Carol Johnston on Diabetes, 29 people were divided into 3 groups.

One-third of the volunteers were type 2 diabetic patients; another one-third were people with signs that they could have diabetes in the future (prediabetic symptoms) while the other third were healthy people.

They were given a vinegar dose before a heavy carbohydrate meal made of bagel, orange juice, and butt.

Some were given meals without vinegar. After a week, they came back for reversed treatment.

Their blood sugar was tested after the meal and was found out that the prediabetic group got the biggest gain as their blood sugar rise after the meal reduced by a whopping 50% compared to those who did not take vinegar with their meal.

The blood glucose for the diabetic group was only 25% better.

Prediabetic people gave lower blood glucose than healthy volunteers when both groups took Vinegar with their meals.

It was found out that this vinegar treatment gave results comparable to popular diabetics' drugs like Metformin.

They got some other unexpected results which was a plus.

Volunteers who used vinegar treatment had a moderate weight loss which is good news.

Now, that we know that those prediabetic volunteers gained more by coming out with lower glucose level, would it not be better to occasionally give oneself a vinegar treatment to prevent diabetes?

Sounds sensible, doesn't it

And what is the dosage?

Two tablespoons of vinegar before a meal, or possibly as a salad dressing.

Or. Apple Cider Vinegar diabetic drink

250 mils of water.
Half cup unfiltered, organic apple juice.
Two teaspoons Apple Cider Vinegar.

Mix and drink on empty stomach in the morning.

38. Diaper Rashes: Smoothen Baby's Skin.

For diaper rashes on your baby, Apple Cider Vinegar comes in handy.

A teaspoon of ACV in a half cup of water is the recipe.

Dab lightly on the rashes on the baby using a towel.

You can be sure the antibacterial substances in ACV will fight the rashes.

Baking soda works as well.

39. Diarrhoea: Stop The Flow.

Diarrhoea often occurs in unexpected places, in the office, in the mall, or at home. Wherever it occurs it is an unpleasant experience.

Diarrhoea is considered a symptom but not a medical condition because it is a way for the body to expel those unwanted substances in the stomach.

This could be caused by partly digested food, parasites, or viruses.

These irritants are expelled from the body as diarrhoea.

Oftentimes, Diarrhoea will subside on its own but it's better stopped to prevent loss of too much water.

Of course, there are OTC medications but as usual, it may be replacing one problem with another.

Apple Cider Vinegar is our friend, so we go to him for help.

One cup of warm water
Two tablespoon Apple Cider Vinegar

Mix properly and drink over a time of about twenty minutes and hourly until the symptom disappears. Just the one preparation.

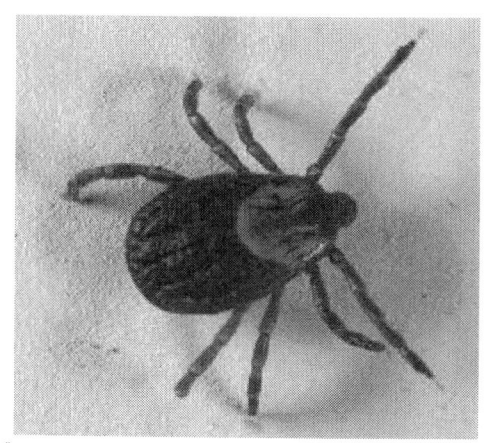

40. Dog Ticks: Dogs Don't Like Them.

It would have been surprising if Apple Cider Vinegar has no effect on Dog ticks and pests with its acidic and antibacterial properties.

To fight off ticks on your dog, put an equal volume of Apple Cider Vinegar and water in a spray bottle, and use to spray your dog. This kills the ticks.

You can also use this solution now and then, say once a week, to keep the ticks away from infecting the dog.

41. Douching: Keep Female Down Clean And Fresh.
To get a healthier Virginia, douche it, and bath with Apple Cider Vinegar regularly.

Apple Cider Vinegar keeps women troubles away.

Douche mixture.

Two tablespoons of Apple Cider Vinegar
One litre of warm water, distilled water is better.

Use the mixture for douching.

If you have discharges you may do this twice daily.

For a bath, add two cups ACV to bathwater.

For a Sitz bath, which is the bathing of the area around the anus, the vulva, the rectum, and the scrotum: use one cup of Apple Cider Vinegar in enough warm water.

42. Dry Hair: Make Hairs Lush Again.
On weekly basis, apply olive oil or castor oil to hair. Add Apple Cider Vinegar to your scalp as in under dandruff.

Leave for from thirty minutes to three hours before shampooing.

Lush hair.

43. Ear Drops: Clean The Cochlea Dirt.

Apple cider vinegar is very effective as ear drops. Mix 50/50 ACV and warm water.

Put in a dropper bottle and use to apply about five drops in each ear one at a time.

Cover the ear with cotton wool and lean on the other side to allow the solution to enter and do its work.

Repeat for the second ear. Hydrogen Peroxide works too.

See swimmer ear.

44. Eczema: Embarrassing.

Eczema is a discomforting skin condition existing as patches and discoloration of the skin.

In this group, you have dyshidrotic eczema, atopic dermatitis, and contact dermatitis.

Eczema is said to be triggered by allergen which makes medics classify it as an immune disorder.

There is no known orthodox cure for Eczema but there are many proprietary products in the market which claim to treat this condition but more often than not it will reappear.

There are natural treatments for eczema though and Apple Cider Vinegar comes top on the list

It has been found that ACV with its antibacterial, antifungal and antiviral properties are effective on Eczema as it kills the bacteria and dries off.

All you need is two cups of Apple Cider Vinegar in warm water to give you a warm bath to fight off the disease and moisturize the skin.

You may soak a towel in the warm solution and apply it to the place for thirty minutes. Repeat regularly until it clears off.

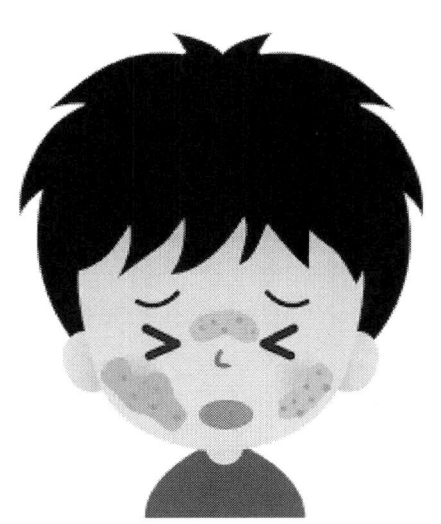

Alternatively, mix ACV with sulphur ointment and apply directly to the affected area.

Apply on a small portion first and check for skin irritation. If it burns or irritates discontinue.

Apple Cider Vinegar is said to work wonders on babies' skin.

Give your baby a warm Apple Cider Vinegar bath now and then to moisturize the skin and keep eczema away.

You may want to combine this therapy with eczema proprietary products to get eczema out fast.

Wash all used clothes in hot water to prevent reoccurrence.

45. Emphysema: Clear The Air Sacs.

Emphysema and Chronic Obstructive Pulmonary Disease (COPD) is a pulmonary disease where the air sacs in the lungs are stretched and damaged.

The result is difficulty in breathing and chronic cough.

This condition is usually caused by smoking, but it could also be hereditary.

There is no cure. However, if sufferers abstain from smoking the effect will be reduced as further damage to the air sacs will stop.

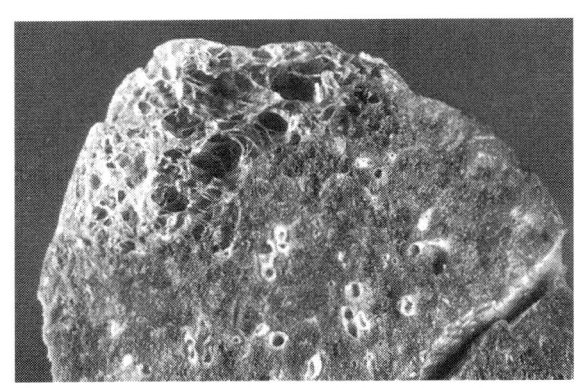

ACV wet press can help in reducing the pains.

Place a thin cloth soaked in Apple Cider Vinegar over the chest. Cover with a wrap and use a hot water flat bottle or hot wrung-out towel to heat the chest area.

Allow the Apple Cider Vinegar to be absorbed by the skin. It will give you some relief.

You can use the same system for throat infection along with gargling. This is also a cool therapy for flu, bronchitis colds, and asthma.

Please see treatments for these ailments elsewhere in this book.

46. Face Toning: Lighter Face Shines Better.

You can make your face lighter with Apple Cider Vinegar.

We will approach this in 2 ways.

1. Two tablespoons of ACV.
Seven tablespoons water.

First, clean your face by washing.

Then apply on the face with cotton wool.

Allow the concentrate to work on the face for 15minutes.

Wash off and dry using a towel.

If your skin is very sensitive dilute with more water

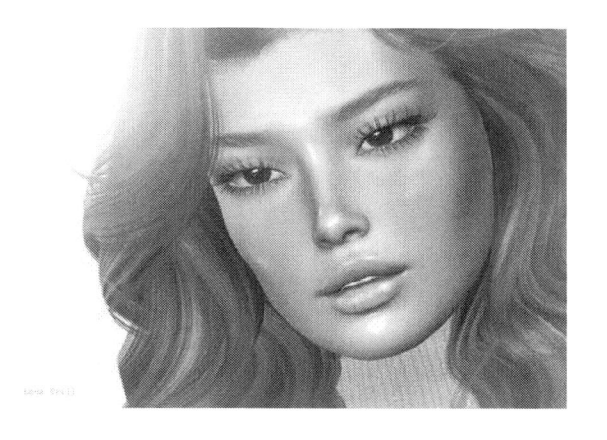

2.A glass of water
Two tablespoons of Apple Cider Vinegar.
One teaspoon of any of these (Rose Essence, Flower Water, Vanilla, Almond Extract.)
Three drops of any essential oil like lavender.
One teaspoon of Horse Chestnut or Witch Hazel

Mix together and apply as 1 above. If your face is not oily, you may not add Witch Hazel

47. Fasting: Body Cleanser.

Fasting is a long-tested and trusted way of cleaning the body.

Many people fast for spiritual purposes but fasting has health benefits and it detoxifies the body.

You may have taken an excess of food, alcohol, or beverages, fasting will flush the remnants out.

Unfortunately, many people dread fasting. They cannot be without food until noon.

Such people will get a helping hand from Apple Cider Vinegar fasting.

ACV helps you during fasting by helping you to absorb minerals in the food already taken before the fast. This makes you full, satisfied, and healthy.

Pioneers of Apple Cider Vinegar fasting have a recipe for ACV fasting.

250 mils of water
Half tablespoon Apple Cider Vinegar.
Half tablespoon lemon juice.
Drink three to four times a day for about a week.

You may increase the ACV to a tablespoon on the third day

Best taken in the morning or at night.

48. Fever Blisters: Ugly Sight, You Don't Want Them.

Fever blisters or Cold sores are blisters you get on the lips or corners of the lips, or inside the mouth and sometimes in the nose when you have had a fever or about to.

These are caused by viruses and Apple Cider Vinegar is known for its antimicrobial and antibacterial properties which make it suitable to deal with the sores.

The treatment removes dead cells and cures the painful sore.

How?

1.   Five mills of ACV in Fifty mills water.

Mix and apply on the sore with cotton wool twice daily.

2.   Mix equal volume of Apple Cider Vinegar and water, apply on the sore for about 10 minutes before removing the blisters carefully with a wet towel.

Please do not use undiluted vinegar as it may burn your skin.

49. Fever: Weakens You, Fight It.

Let us look at it this way.

The apple fruit we eat contains ample vitamins C and E, potassium, and antioxidants among others.

These all combine to have a better functioning lung.

This means the throat is clearer loosening phlegm in the process.

When you spit out phlegm you have a feeling you are getting better.

These constituents can wrestle down the sickness causing pathogens.

Now, if we get these from raw apple fruit, does it not make sense to believe that Apple Cider Vinegar made from apple will help in fighting a cold?

Yes, it does. ACV fights cold and fever.

One-part ACV and two parts water, soak a towel and put it on your forehead or wrap the soles of your feet with the towel. Or do both.

50. Fibres: You Also Need Them.

Fibre is another word for roughages which we get from veggies, fruits, nuts and so on. They are very useful to the body.

There are two types, soluble and insoluble fibres.

Benefits include giving you fullness even with little food, low incidence of sugar spike, and therefore lesser risk of heart disease.

You can get roughages naturally but Apple Cider Vinegar has some fibre in it even though not much.

Apple Cider Vinegar has small amount of fibre which makes it possible to combine with other materials like sorbitol, a sugar alcohol,

Add one to two tablespoon of ACV to a glass of water and drink.

The fibre there gives you some fullness which stops you from bringing in junks in-between meals: a good recipe for weight loss.

51. Flatulence: Ease off the Gas.

Gas and bloating in the alimentary canal is Flatulence and this may be caused by slow digestion and unhealthy food.

Unhealthy food can cause a lot of damage to the food track and the system as a whole.

Whether flatulence is caused by unhealthy food or not, there are many OTC products to treat it.

Some people however prefer the natural way and Apple Cider Vinegar comes in handy here.

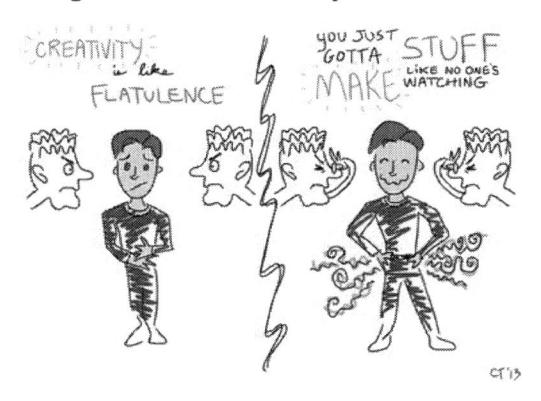

Since ACV has antimicrobial properties, it follows it will kill the bacteria in the alimentary canal, namely the stomach and intestines.

When this happens, Flatulence subsides.

Use a tablespoon of Apple Cider Vinegar in warm water and drink before your next meal. ACV also has enzymes that will aid your digestion.

This is an Apple Cider Vinegar tonic for flatulence.

One Teaspoon of Apple Cider Vinegar.
One cup of water
One teaspoon of honey
One teaspoon of peppermint
Mix and consume once in a day.

52. Fleas Spray: Nuisance Fleas.

Sometimes you see your pet is scratching her body as a result of flies bite. If you have this luck, just invite Apple Cider Vinegar to help you.

Put Equal volume of ACV and water in a spaying bottle and spay the pet's fur. The fleas will die and no more infections.

53. Food Poisoning: Uncomfortable.

Apple Cider Vinegar can help reduce symptoms of food poisoning because it can sooth the lining of the stomach and kill excess bacteria.

Just drink a tablespoon of ACV in a cup of hot water before your meal.

54. Gallbladder: Be Nice to The Flusher.

You know the Liver and the Gallbladder work together to rid the body of toxins and balance the body's ph.

You can therefore see why it becomes imperative to maintain a clean and healthy Gallbladder.

If the flusher is dirty, then it is hampered in doing its job.

Apple Cider Vinegar gallbladder flush comes in handy here.

How do you do the ACV flush?

Fill the normal glass cup to 66% level with organic apple juice and top with organic olive oil and one teaspoon of organic Apple Cider Vinegar, not concentrate, but Briggs ACV if possible.

Drink three times the first day and two times the second day.

You may do this twice a year.

Flushing your system like this prevents gallstones that are caused by too much bilirubin (a yellowish substance formed when red blood cells break down) in the bile.

Another cause of gallbladder stones is when the Gallbladder is not strong enough to dissolve the cholesterol produced by the liver which may later crystallize to gallbladder stones. Flushing the gallbladder also prevents this.

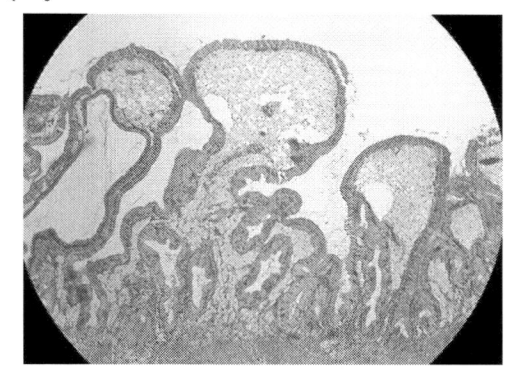

Warning. Diabetic Patients Should Not Do This Flush.

55. Gerd.
(Gastroesophageal Reflux Disease)

See: Acid Reflux, Heart Burn & GERD

56. Gingivitis: Protect Your Teeth.

Inflammation of the gum and at times the inside of the mouth is called gingivitis which may not be harmful on its own but when not treated for a long time may lead to a more serious medical condition which may lead to loss of teeth.

The normal treatment is to kill off the bacteria causing this infection and as usual, there are thousands out there which may be expensive, besides the possibility of side effects.

We can invite our friend Apple Cider Vinegar with its acid and pH balancing property.

Gargle with 50/50m solution of Apple Cider Vinegar and water for thirty seconds in the morning before brushing your teeth.

Spit out the gargle.

57. Hair Conditioner: Easy To Make.

You could use Apple Cider Vinegar as a Hair conditioner.

Recipe.

One Tablespoon honey.
Two tablespoon ACV.
Two cups of water.

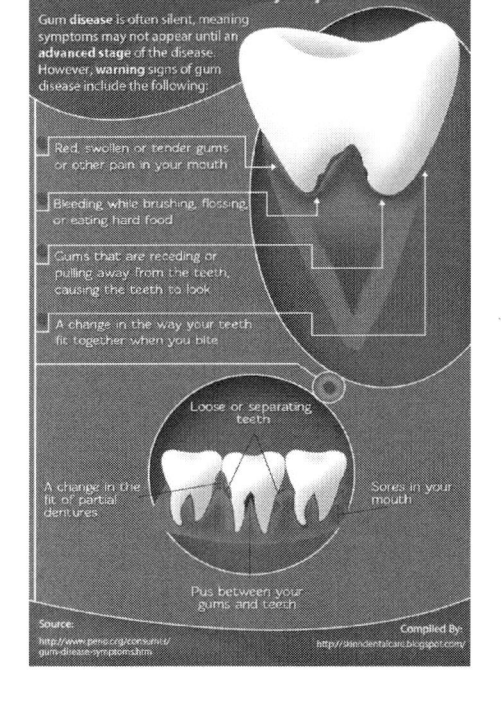

Mix thoroughly in a bowl and apply on the hair tips after shampooing making sure it does not get to the scalp. No rinsing.

Alternatively, you may let it get to the scalp but rinse later.

58. Hair Follicle Growth: Possible.

For where the hairs are thinning out, apply two tablespoons of Apple Cider Vinegar and cayenne powder (a pinch) one hour prior to shampooing.

Do not let it drop into the eyes

On the bald area, mix royal jelly cap and a teaspoon of ACV and pat on bald areas.

Leave overnight.

ACV will not revive a bald head, but baldness may be delayed or hampered when ACV is applied when the hairs start to thin out.

As you will find out elsewhere ACV does a tremendous job in making the hair and scalp happy.

59. Hair Frizz: Tame Them.

Apple cider vinegar is a weak straight-chain hydroxyl acid. Remember the properties?

When you apply ACV directly on the hair, it will help subdue frizzy hairs, removing residues that had dulled the hair leaving them now shinning.

60. Hair Rinse.

Mixture: This Is It

Keep this solution in the shower to use.

To a litre of water add two cups of Apple Cider Vinegar. Mix well and keep in a plastic bottle for hair rinse.

61. Hair: Shine Your Hair.

Apple Cider Vinegar will make your hair shine and also remove the flakes leaving your hair soft.

Being acidic, it removes the build-up of dirt and also balances your hair ph.

Mix a hundred mills of ACV and a litre of water to rinse the hair thoroughly after shampooing, then rinse with ordinary water again.

One hour after, wash your hair normally.

See Dandruff.

62. Hard water: Remove The Minerals Build-Up.

Hard water is caused by mineral build-up which you can treat with Apple Cider Vinegar or lemon/lime to soften.

Mix one tablespoon of ACV with three cups of pure water and use the solution on your hair.

Leave the solution in the hair for about five minutes then wash off thoroughly.

63. Head Ache And Migraines: Signs Of Deeper Trouble?

Many people blame their headaches for the failure of many organs in the body.

Organs such as the liver, the heart, the kidney, the stomach, the sinuses, etc. They may be right.

Headache and pains are the red lights given by mother nature to warn that something is wrong deep down.

Headache is a signal giving by the body that there is a problem somewhere and there are thousands of ways this problem could come.

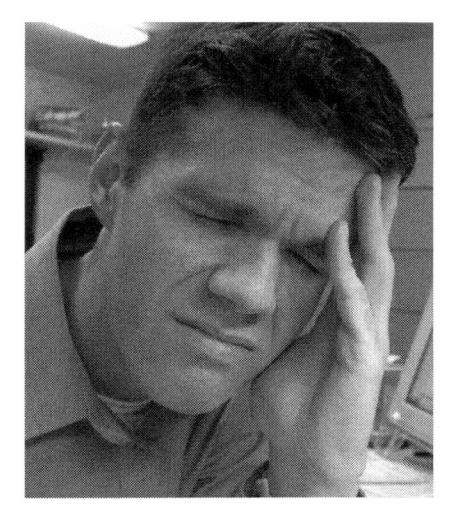

So a headache could be a result of an organ not functioning properly and could be the reason why the organ is malfunctioning.

Stress, dehydration, muscle tension, poor diet, sinus pressure, and mere cold could cause headaches but whatever the cause, it is very discomforting.

You see, our relationship with others does affect our health.

Annoying subordinates, a problematic child, or a nagging spouse could throw you into hours of thinking that may end in a headache.

Whatever the type, it should be taken seriously.

The worst type of headache is one that has developed into migraines which makes the sufferer feel as if the head is splitting into two.

We will deal with headaches in three ways.

1. Apple Cider Vinegar vapour. Add two tablespoons of ACV to 2 cups of water you have brought to boil. Remove the container, bend over it, and inhale the vapour deep about 6 times.

2. Do vinegar compresses. See Emphysema

3. One tablespoon Apple Cider Vinegar, one cup decaffeinated tea, Mix, and drink hourly.

Most importantly, eat and live healthily.

64. Heartburn: Fire In The Thoracic Cavity.

See: Acid Reflux, Heartburn, and GERD

65. Hiccups: You Don't Need Them.

Repetitive spasm of the diaphragm leading to the closing of the vocal cords is believed to be responsible for the hiccup sound which could be very discomforting.

It is harmless, so we think, and lasts momentarily.

However, there have been cases of it lasting for days or even weeks.

No medication for this condition as it vamooses with some bouts of water but Apple Cider Vinegar can drive it away faster.

Mix one tablespoon each of ACV and water. Sip in-between.

66. Haemorrhoids: Stop It In Its Track.

When you apply pressure on veins during movements of the bowel, there are chances that the veins will be swollen. When this happens, the condition is referred to as Hemorrhoids.

It is a common condition around the rectum and the anus, which could be internal or external.

When internal haemorrhoid bulges outward (prolapses) through the anus, it brings with it mucus that can make more severe the itches and irritation that usually accompany this condition

There are home remedies to wrestle down Hemorrhoids and happily enough organic Apple Cider Vinegar Is one of them at the top there.

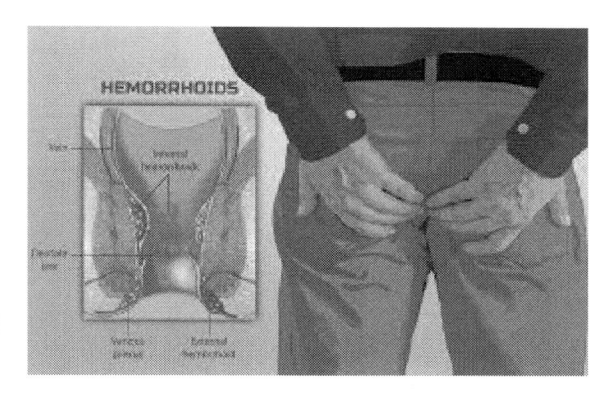

ACV being astringent, because of Acetic acid presence will shrink skin tissues. We know that.

This coupled with her antibacterial property makes Apple Cider Vinegar a top candidate to treat haemorrhoids.

Recipes.

1. Use diluted Apple Cider Vinegar directly on your Hemorrhoid for relief. Apply 50/50 ACV and Water directly on Hemorrhoid.

2. Alternatively, you could have an Apple Cider Vinegar warm bath in your tub. Two cups of ACV in warm water in the tub will do.

Just soak your body in the solution for about thirty minutes to get relief. Take a shower afterward to rinse your body.

3. You could also use frozen Apple Cider Vinegar. You freeze your ACV in a tray in your freezer and break into cubes.

This gives you a cooling effect and relief from itches and pain.

4. There is also an ACV drink for you. A tablespoon of Apple Cider Vinegar in water to drink and drive Hemorrhoids away.

67. Herpes Virus: Trouble for Virus.

One part of Apple Cider Vinegar in three parts of water to be applied directly to the area with Herpes.

You will get a positive result.

We should not be surprised that Apple Cider Vinegar treats herpes virus because Apple Cider Vinegar has antiviral and anti-inflammatory properties.

68. Hives: Get Relief.

Hives, also known as Urticaria is a sudden outbreak of plaques or bumps on the skin appearing in red or pale colors.

Usually, it comes with itching but at times it may burn or sting.

For relief of Hives, take a bath of ACV

Add some drops of Apple Cider Vinegar to your bathwater.

Alternatively, dab the area with a mixture of Apple Cider Vinegar and water.

You can also have a bath of water with some quantity of Baking Soda to get relief.

69. Hypertension: You Can Avoid It.

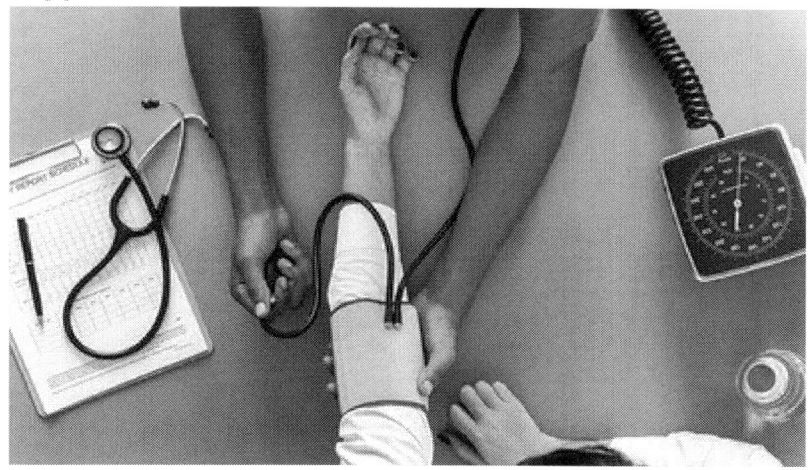

Imagine your water pump pumping mud instead of water.

It goes on pumping until it becomes unbearable for it to continue because of the viscosity of the mud.

With time it stops. It cannot pump again.

The heart is like the pump. I dare say the engineers who made the water pump copied God because if you have ever opened up a water pump and compare it to the heart, they are very similar.

The heart is responsible for pumping the blood through the arteries, blood vessels, and capillaries.

This is a very serious job which becomes more difficult when the blood thickens as a result of it being clogged with fat.

When the blood thickens, it becomes more difficult for the heart to pump and as it forces itself to pump, the blood pressure increases and hypertension occurs.

Acids from natural foods and animal protein help to make the blood thinner for the blood to circulate freely and among the acid-producing substances is our friend Apple Cider Vinegar.

What causes the blood to thicken? Bad eating habits, too much fat, excessive stress even though some could be genetic

Drink a mixture of one cup of water and half tablespoon ACV about 4 times a day without food but with about 8 glasses of water should bring the pressure down.

We must learn to eat healthily, a healthy lifestyle, cut down on fats, caffeinated drinks, sugar, salt, and junk food.

Do enough exercise.

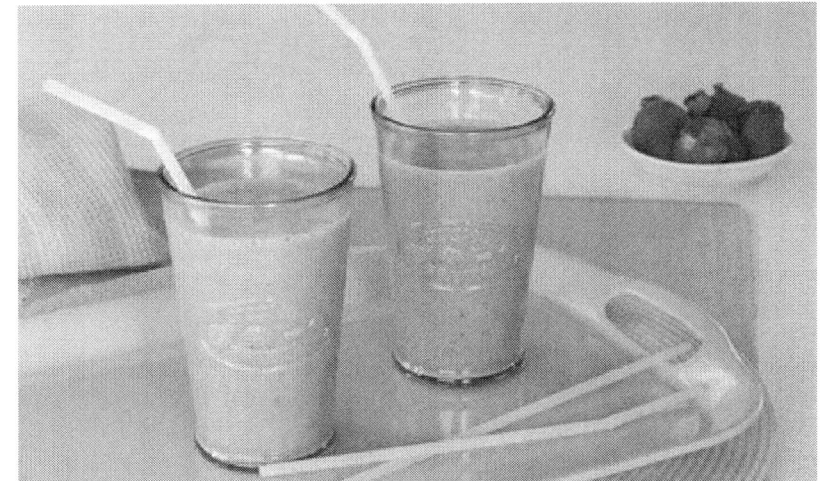

70. Immunity Booster: Spike Your Immunity.

Apple Cider Vinegar is acidic with a high concentration of vitamins, acids, and fibres which are known to boost immunity, breaking down the pathogens that cause loss of immunity.

No wonder during COVAD-19 in 2019 and 2020, vitamin C and vinegar were mentioned prominently.

The ACV detox we are going to make here may be used for a lot of medical conditions which may necessitate us referring to it in this book now and then.

The detox immunes your system reduces your appetite and therefore calorie intake while the bacteria in Apple Cider Vinegar aids digestion which results in bloat reduction and flat tummy.

Recipe.

Ingredients.

1. Apple Cider Vinegar.
2. Almighty Ginger
3. Lemon
4. Raw Honey
5. Cinnamon

Note. Your ACV must have the mother.

We talked about this in 'differences between Apple Cider Vinegar and white vinegar'. So your Apple Cider Vinegar must have the mother which you notice at the bottom of the bottle as a cob-web like sediment.

This will be raw, unfiltered, and undiluted Apple Cider Vinegar. Get Bragg Apple Cider Vinegar if you can.

Your almighty ginger is better raw but if you cannot get it raw, you may use the powdered Ginger.

Lemon must be raw too to get undiluted vitamin C for immunity boosting. You remember Vitamin C and Lemon are mentioned prominently in treatment for Covid-19.

Your honey has to be pure as against Honey made from Sugar cane. We know of several uses of Horney including treating sore throat and burns.

Raw honey has antioxidant properties that help to build the immune system. Besides, it gives the sour taste of ACV some sweetness.

Who knows we may come to write on medicinal uses of Horney one day.

Let me whet your appetite a bit before the book is written.

Besides sore throat healing and antioxidant properties, pure honey helps in healing burns and wounds, aids digestion, smoothens the skin and also has antibacterial properties.

I have a recipe of Ginger, turmeric, and honey that gives me energy on and out of bed.

Cinnamon has antiviral and antibacterial properties in addition to being an analgesic and anti-inflammatory agent.

These are good properties needed in the preparation of an immunity-boosting detox.

Preparation

1. 300cm3 of hot water

2. One tablespoon of grated ginger or a quarter teaspoon of powdered ginger

3. One tablespoon of Apple Cider Vinegar with mother.

4. A pinch of cinnamon

5. Half a cup of lemon juice.

6. Raw honey to reduce the sour taste of Apple Cider Vinegar.

Mix Cinnamon and grated ginger, add the Apple Cider Vinegar and then water (hot), add the lemon juice and the Honey and drink.

If you want to spice it up, you may change lemon juice to orange juice, add some drops of cherry juice, mint leaves, or muddles berries.

The hot water may be replaced by sparkling water aka carbonated water.

Drink on empty stomach before breakfast and before dinner for the best result. It will stop many ailments in their track.

If you want more quantity you can increase the ingredients in the ration above.

WARNING.

Do Not Drink Raw Apple Cider Vinegar straight, Always Dilute It With Water

71. Infections: Stop Them in Their Track.

Apple Cider Vinegar may not cure UTI (Urinary Tract Infection) completely but it may prevent it and don't we all say prevention is better than cure?

Staphylococcus Aures and Eshnerica Coli are bacterias causing infection in the urinary tract.

They exist naturally in the tract especially the bowel but they can cause infections.

Our friend ACV prevents them from doing any damage.

One Tablespoon Apple Cider Vinegar, 250mils of water, mix together and consume in three potions a day.

Adding a teaspoon of honey to the mixture does not hurt.

Drink plenty of water.

72. Inflammation: Not Good Anywhere.

The body responds to toxins build up in tissues by getting inflamed.

What we eat can curtail inflammation while some foods may aid it.

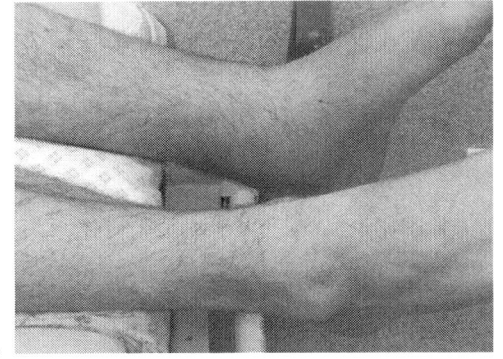

Food with a high content of toxins can aggravate inflammation while food rich in nutrients can curtail inflammation

Drink a mixture of one cup of water and one tablespoon Apple Cider Vinegar.

73. Inner Ecosystem Balancing: Moving Toward Equilibrium.

The body normally tries to maintain a state of equilibrium medically called a state of homeostasis.

To do this, the body system has to balance the Acid-base ratio to get a pH of between 7.34 and 7.45. ACV helps to maintain this.

Too acidic system leads to mucous production and loss of energy and reduction in resistance to infection and other ailments

A solution of 50/50 water and Apple Cider Vinegar will do.

Drink.

74. Insomnia: Sleeping Is Your Right.

Insomnia could range from sleep disruptions to total sleeplessness and could be caused by many factors including stress, sickness, side effects of medication, unhealthy lifestyle, and eating habits. etc.

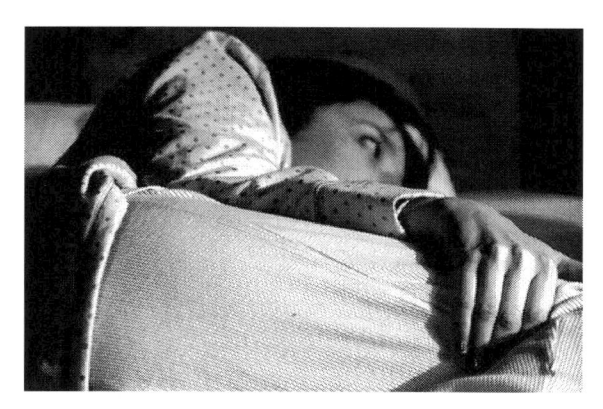

Insomnia could be corrected by eating nutrient-filled foods and a better lifestyle but unfortunately, many people result to medications including sleeping pills which may, unfortunately, come with its own problems.

Wise people help themselves with doses of Apple Cider Vinegar,

One tablespoon of ACV, with honey as a spice and a cup of warm water or non-stimulant organic tea.

Drink before bed and sleep tight.

75. Interstitial Cystitis: Flay The Cramps and Pains.

We already know about the flushing ability of Apple Cider Vinegar which we deploy in cleansing the liver and bladder.

We also know about bacteria cystitis; therefore, we should not be surprised that Apple Cider Vinegar cures interstitial cystitis.

Interstitial cystitis is inflammation of the walls of the intestine which gives the sufferer pains and cramps similar to what we have in bacteria cystitis.

Many people who had suffered intestinal pains got relief by using ACV.

Recipe.

Two teaspoons of Apple Cider Vinegar
A cup of water
Some drops of honey.

Mix thoroughly and drink twice per day.

See bacteria cystitis.

76. Iron absorption: Iron for Strength.

Add two tablespoons of Apple Cider Vinegar to drinking water and drink before each meal to help abstract iron from the food you eat into the system.

Spinach is an example of iron-containing foods that you may eat after the ACV drink.

This improves your iron bioavailability in addition to spiking your hydrochloric acid level and aiding digestion.

You may mix your Apple Cider Vinegar with squeezed lemon and drink before meals.

77. Irritable Bowel syndrome: Discomforting.

Irritable Bowel Syndrome happens largely in the large intestine as a result of incomplete digestion and it comes with abdominal pains, cramps, bloating, and even constipation and diarrhea.

Not so much a serious problem as many can manage it by living and eating healthily.

More serious cases could be treated with medication but Apple Cider Vinegar helps.

The following food may cause IBS. Food full of fibers, fatty and oily foods, carbonated drinks, and a large meal at a time. Do not forget chocolate, caffeinated drinks, and alcohol, they may cause IBS.

For prevention of IBS, mix two cups of water and one tablespoon ACV. Drink by sips before a meal.

To treat IBS, mix one cup of water with three teaspoons of Apple Cider Vinegar. Sip over a period of about thirty minutes.

78. Joint Pain: Watch It.

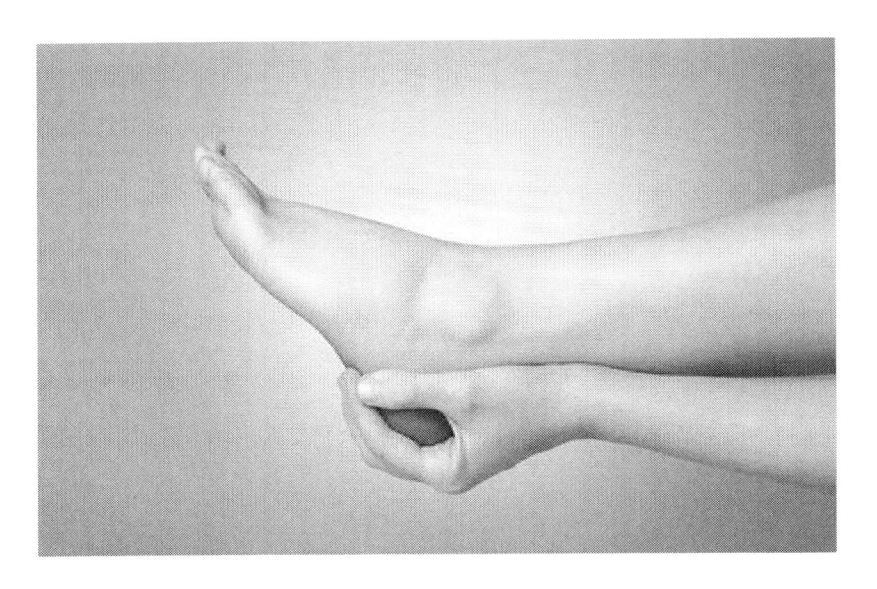

See Rheumatoid Arthritis

79. Kidney: Clean The Body's Second Most Important Factory.

It is believed that vinegar helps to rid the body of toxins and minerals which may lead to kidney stones.

Apple Cider Vinegar has a cleansing effect on the liver and the kidney.

The acetic acid in ACV flushes the kidney and also helps to reduce pains caused by the stones.

To 200mls of clean or distilled water, add two tablespoons of Apple Cider Vinegar plus one teaspoon honey.

Drink in two to three portions daily.

You may want to refer to Gallbladder flush.

Drink plenty of water daily. You cannot over drink water. It helps greatly in body cleansing.

80. Laryngitis: Let's Get Melodious.

When the larynx is inflamed resulting in loss of voice or voice huskiness accompanied by hard breathing and cough, that is Laryngitis.

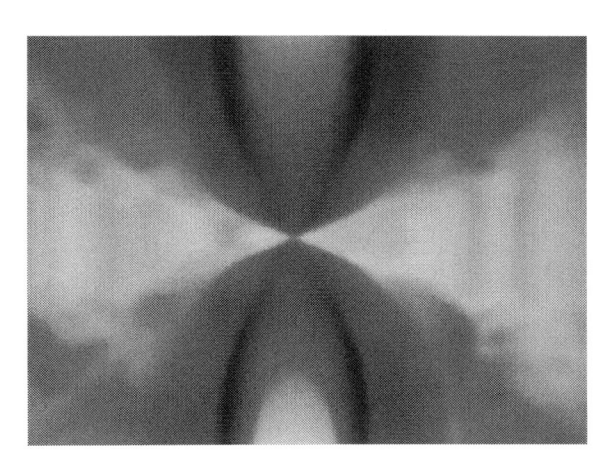

Do not bother, Apple Cider Vinegar will help. Organic ACV is a great tormentor of mucus and germs attacking the throat.

Get a glass of water, add 2 tablespoon of organic Apple Cider Vinegar plus a sweetener such as honey (one tablespoon). Drink twice per day and watch your condition improve.

Or, gargle with a solution of two teaspoons of Apple Cider Vinegar to two glasses of warm water. Do three mouthfuls every hour until you get relief.

Don't swallow the gargled solution, spit it out each time.

You could also do saltwater gaggle. Just add a little Apple Cider Vinegar to the saltwater.

I have done this several times with good results.

What of ACV wet press under Emphysema? It's an alternative therapy too.

For Laryngitis, many performing musicians turn to Apple Cider Vinegar therapy.

81. Leg cramps: Free The Legs.

Too much physical exertion, dehydration, and poor circulation may give you, leg cramps among other issues.

There are OTC creams, drugs, and anti-inflammatory drugs to give you relief which may be temporary.

Get some honey and dissolve in it two teaspoons of Apple Cider Vinegar and drink. You have just taken a solution to give you relief from leg cramps.

This solution and mustard or pickle juice are common with athletes.

Mix two cups water, one tablespoon Apple Cider Vinegar. Drink twice daily until it subsides.

This is another one. Do an Apple Cider Vinegar tub bath. A cup of Apple Cider Vinegar in a full tub for a bath.

Or dampen a towel with Apple Cider Vinegar and apply directly to the cramped area.

Support with reflexology for quicker relief.

82. Lice: Frustrating Scratching In The Public.

Lice in the head can be frustrating. You keep scratching the head and they are easily transferrable especially among children and in crowded places.

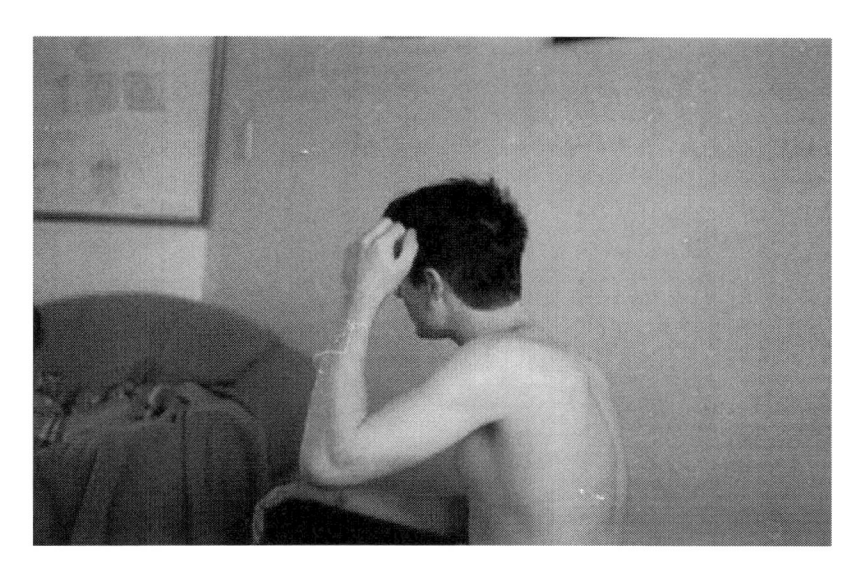

You can deal with them medically but why that, when you have Apple Cider Vinegar.

Give the head an ACV treatment by applying the Apple Cider Vinegar solution on the hair. Cover the hair with a cap for about 4 hours after which you wash and comb finely to remove dead lice and the eggs.

83. Listerine Foot Bath: Clear Off The Dead Cells.

Listerine is the brand name for a mild antiseptic named after Sir Lister normally used for cleansing.

Surprisingly, it combines well with vinegar to remove dead cells on the feet and fingers.

This is understandable as Benzoic acid the main component of Listering has exfoliating properties that work well with Acetic acid the main component of Vinegar to see the dead cells off and kill the fungus.

Get enough water to cover your feet in a bowl, add enough quantity of Apple Cider Vinegar and some leistering solution and sink your feet in the solution for about 30minutes.

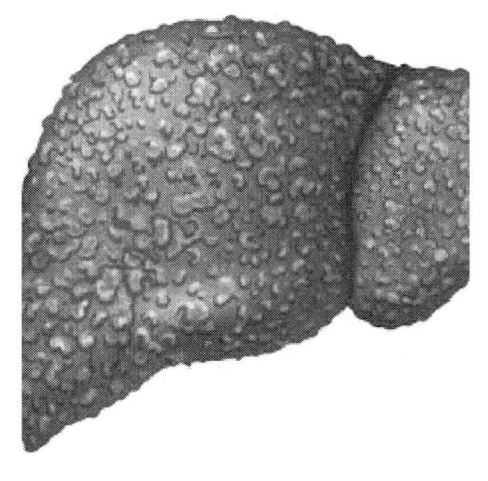

Wash with warm water or scrub gently if you like and dry up.

Watch as the fungus and dead cells clear of.

84. Liver, Hepatitis: Caring For The Body's First Giant Factory.

The human liver is a giant factory manufacturing bile for digestion and also a great filterer of toxins and waste from the blood. Besides those, it energizes you.

You need to keep your liver toxin-free and healthy for you to have a healthy life. Some people believe the liver is the next most important organ in the body, next to the heart

To help the liver you have to eat healthily, take minimal alcohol, eat fruits, and run away from toxic foods.

Doctors have not confirmed that ACV can help in the treatment of Hepatitis C. It is neither here nor there. However, there are some who can swear that it helps.

However, with the properties of Apple Cider Vinegar, it seems it may help in detoxifying the liver, boosting immunity, and reducing inflammation which in turn helps to improve the symptoms of hepatitis C patients.

This is explainable as ACV has detoxifying properties which help in the promotion of circulation in the Liver.

By so doing, Apple Cider Vinegar helps in removing deadly toxins that tend to build in weak livers.

Inflammation is one of the causes of hepatitis C and if it is agreed that ACV has anti-inflammatory properties, then it could help in treating hepatitis c according to the American Liver Foundation.

So, can you use Apple Cider Vinega for a damaged liver?

Like we said above, it's neither here nor there as no two individuals have the same medical conditions, and talking to a doctor about it may be the best course.

This is a liver cleansing tonic.

Two teaspoons Apple Cider Vinegar, one cup water, half teaspoon raw honey. Drink two to three times daily.

85. Malnutrition: Beef Up A Little.

Malnutrition is basically caused by unhealthy eating. Mal is bad, therefore malnutrition is bad nutrition.

People suffering from malnutrition lack energy, vigour and the do power. Their foods lack the necessary vitamins and nutrients to give them a sound body

Potassium is a vital mineral which helps in regulating fluid balance and nerve signs and muscle contraction. Enough

Potassium in the system prevents high blood pressure and stroke.

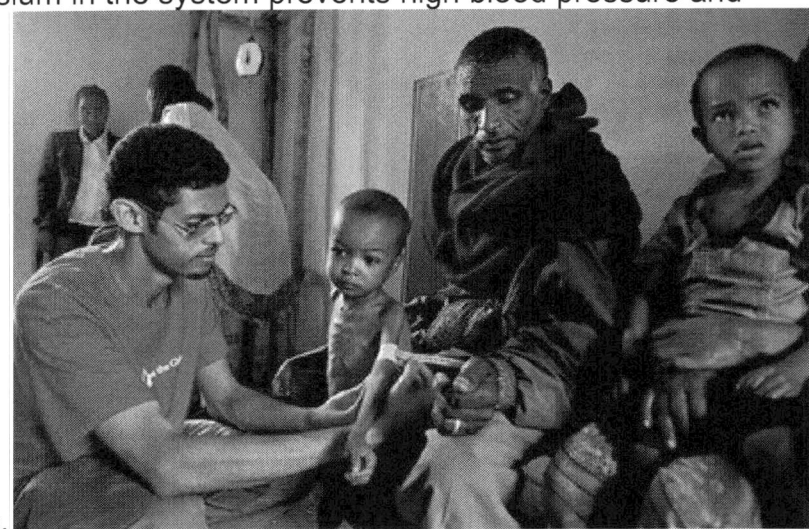

Unfortunately, many food items do not have potassium in enough quantity which makes us look for alternatives to energize us.

Some of us go for caffeinated junks, cola, drugs, and things like these which give us temporary strength and vigour.

They all have their side effects but what do we get when we eat apple?

. "An apple a day keeps the doctor away," Apple is the food of life and it has enough potassium.

And Apple Cider Vinegar is made from natural apple.

Does it not make sense that a drink of Apple Cider Vinegar a day will be good for people suffering from malnutrition?

Yes, it does, so go for ACV tonic to treat malnutrition

86. Mentally Handicapped: They Could Be Helped.

Potassium deficiency makes people senile. Several years ago, one of the pioneers of CAM took in three mentally handicapped kids into their house.

They were given three Apple Cider Vinegar drink three times a day with doses of multivitamins supplements particularly those containing vitamin-3.

One teaspoon of ACV and one teaspoon of raw honey. Mix in a glass of distilled water and drink three times a day.

After three weeks, the kids became more mentally alert.

Apple Cider Vinegar is the liquid of life. Use it for brain development.

See senility.

87. Morning sickness: Sign Of Bundle Of Joy.

Apple Cider Vinegar has a lot of components that are very beneficial to both mom and baby.

It has vitamins A, B, C, and E. It has minerals like Potassium, Magnesium, fibres, and enzymes which are good for mother and baby.

Apple Cider Vinegar also regulates the body pH, improves digestion while it fights constipation.

Now, pregnancy is one experience only a mother can describe. A bulging tummy, a moving baby in the womb, and the feeble kicks.

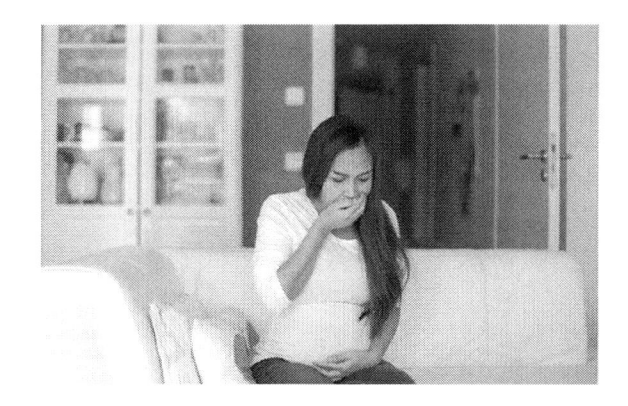

Accompanying this experience is the nauseating and even vomiting that goes with it.

It is called morning sickness never mind that it can occur at any time of the day.

You may want to subdue this with drugs, but why when you have Apple Cider Vinegar?

Half tablespoon ACV, two cups water, a small quantity (a quarter) of peeled Ginger. Sip a little at a time over one hour by which time you should have relief.

88. Morning Smoothes: Best Way To Take Off.

A great way to start a day is to have a Smoothie and the better way to do it is to use a recipe with our friend Apple Cider Vinegar.

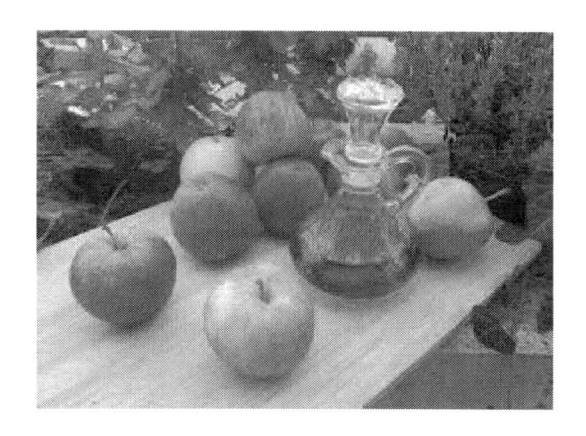

Blend the following thoroughly and drink.

Ingredients:

Half a cup of water.

One packet of sip organic Apple Cider Vinegar.

One Cup of frozen mixed berries.

One peeled banana.

Half cup yogurt.

Half cup ice.

Mix and drink

89. Muscle Stiffness: Supple Muscles Work Best.

Stiffness of the muscle is caused by a build-up of Lactic Acid and it causes pain in body areas such as the back, neck, legs, butts, and arms.

Usually with muscle stiffness, when you stretch the muscles, the physical exercise allows the body to release the Lactic acid into the system to be flushed out.

This gives you relief but some people would prefer to use medication.

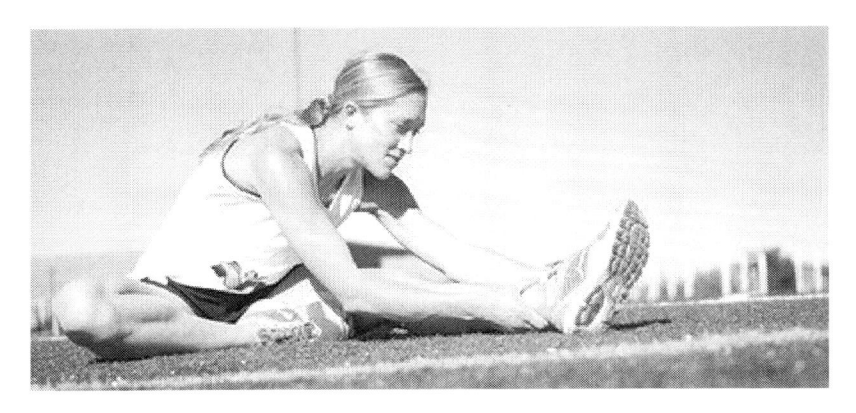

Why expending scarce resources when our friend Apple Cider Vinegar can help?

ACV as you know contains Enzymes, Acetic Acid, minerals, and vitamins to fight the Lactic Acid into the system to be flushed out.

You can approach this in any of these three ways.

Apple Cider Vinegar Drink

Two Teaspoons of Apple Cider Vinegar.

One cup of water.

Mix and drink.

Apple Cider Vinegar Bath

For a soothing bath, soak yourself in a tub of water which has been added two cups of ACV.

Stay in the bath for about 30 minutes.

It is enough time for the system to get rid of Lactic Acid and other toxins.

Hot Apple Cider Vinegar Pressing.

Half cup Apple Cider Vinegar

One cup of warm water.

Soak a towel and squeeze out excess water and press the damp warm towel on the affected areas for about 15 minutes and get relief.

90. Nail Fungus: Kill Them.

By now, we know Apple Cider Vinegar has both anti-fungal and antibacterial properties that qualify it to treat fungi infection including nail fungus.

Besides these properties, ACV also has vitamins and minerals which help in making the nails finer.

There are OTC products you can buy but you are better off with Apple Cider Vinegar treatment.

The Drink.

One Tablespoon of Apple Cider Vinegar.
One cup of water.
Mix to drink for cure and prevention drinking two or three times in a day.

Direct Application.

Soak the nails in lightly diluted Apple Cider Vinegar for about 20 minutes every two hours.

ACV penetrates the pores and kills the fungus.

91. Nasal Wash: For Free Nasal Passage.

Making The solution.

Two teaspoons of Apple Cider Vinegar.
Two glasses of warm water.

Sniff the warm solution up your nostril rolling your head backward, sideways, lean over and blow out the mucus.

Do this two times daily until the nasal passage is clear.

You can sip some juice in between. Good for the body.

This solution can also be used as a throat gargle to fight sore throat and Laryngitis.

Please do not swallow the gargle solution because Apple Cider Vinegar would have extracted some toxins that should not go into your stomach.

Spit out the gargle solution.

You may want to see Laryngitis.

92. Nausea And Vomiting: Irritating.

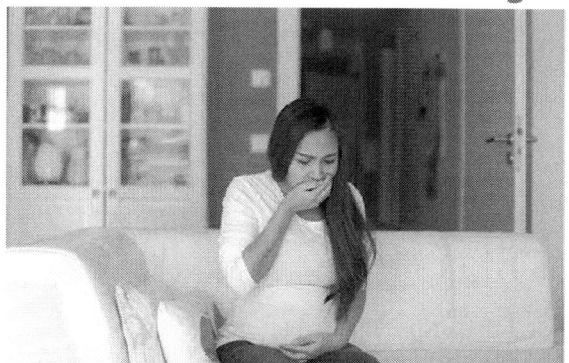

When you are nauseated your stomach is telling you there is something in there making it uncomfortable.

The best solution is to get that thing out by vomiting.

You can do this by drinking a glass of water with a small quantity of Apple Cider Vinegar, regurgitate until the stomach is empty.

It may be necessary to induce vomiting by pressing the end of the tongue in the throat while leaning over the bowl.

It is wise to throw out anything causing stomach upset.

However, if you do not want to vomit you can rely on the antimicrobial property of ACV to prevent vomiting and nausea.

A teaspoon of both honey and Apple Cider Vinegar in 250 mils of water will do.

Sip in small bits throughout the day and see how it calms down your stomach cramps.

Replacing Apple Cider Vinegar with Baking soda gives relief too, but please don't use both Apple Cider Vinegar and Baking Soda together.

93. Nerve Pains (Sciatic Nerve Pain): Free The Nerves.

The Solution

Three litres of warm /hot water

250 mils of Apple Cider Vinegar

A quarter cup of Epsom salt

Mix together.

Soak feet into the solution for thirty minutes.

Remove your feet and dry up.

Wrap in a warm towel.

The next morning Keep the feet warm with socks.

If it affects the upper side of the leg, you may increase the volume of the warm water, ACV, and Epsom salt accordingly.

Do Apple Cider Vinegar press if it occurs further up like the bottom area.

Nerve pain is gone.

94. Nosebleeds: Embarrassment In The Public.

A towel soaked in Apple Cider Vinegar stops bleeding and possible infection.

For years ACV has been used for healing burns, bites, cuts, and so on.

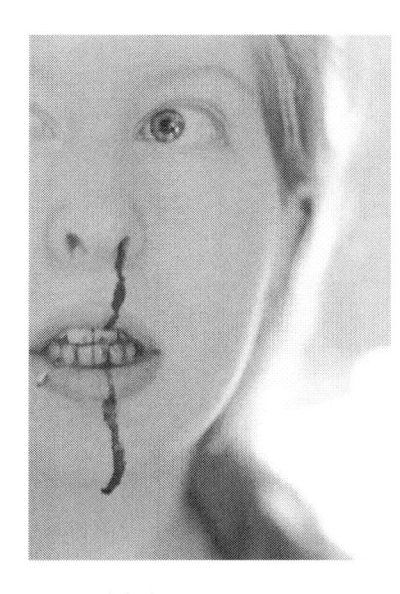

For Nosebleeds insert soaked wool or gauze in the nose.

Relax on a chair, lean forward for 10 minutes breathing through the mouth.

You may want to press the nostril together to congeal the blood and clean later.

Ingest some tabs of vitamins K and C.

As nosebleeds are usually caused by dehydration, you will need to drink sufficient water. You cannot over drink water.

95. Obesity: Burn Off the Fat.

As we are writing this, billions of dollars are spent on weight loss in Europe and America.

Thirty percent of Americans are fighting obesity which is why it is not surprising that a newbie in internet marketing will choose the weight loss niche.

And he will make money.

Most of the time, the wonder recipes dished out don't work. They give you some complicated recipes which get you pissed off trying to put together.

I know because I have travelled the road before. Thanks to ACV.

There is no miracle to weight loss. It needs discipline which starts with a reduction in food intake and the type of food you eat.

ACV is no magic liquid that will burn the fats overnight but it helps you fight obesity drastically.

ACV drinks, with average calorie intake and enough good exercise, will trim the waist and burn the fats.

Two teaspoons plus honey and a glass of distilled water is the drink. Drink daily.

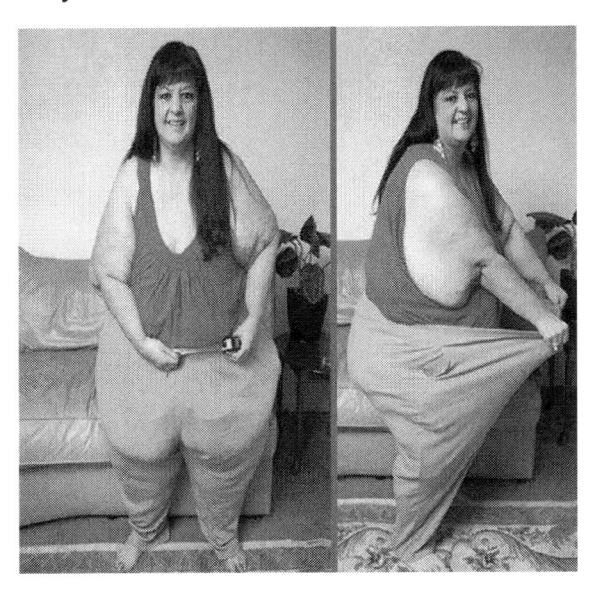

As said earlier, with this Apple Cider Vinegar drink, you must reduce your intake of calories and do some exercises.

Do away with all processed food, sugar, beverages, and dairy products.

Instead, go for organic fruits; raw nuts, raw salads; and seeds; and the likes.

Massages also add some weight loss benefits to the recipe.

96. Parasitic Infections: Stop Them.

Pets, especially dogs may get infested with parasites such as ringworm, hookworm, and even tapeworms.

Preventing them from getting inside the dog may be the best practice as it is a bit difficult to treat.

Make sure you add about 5mills (a teaspoon) of Apple Cider Vinegar in the dogs drinking water on a daily basis.

This will save you sizeable money to buy proprietary products later if infected.

You may use this recipe to treat internal parasites for both humans and dogs.

- One teaspoon of Apple Cider Vinegar with the mother.
- 130mils water.
- One teaspoon honey.
- Squeeze out the content of one lime.

Mix together and drink. For your dog, you can give him small portion of the solution.

Although ACV is beneficial against parasites, but it should not replace de-worming using proprietary products when your pets had already gotten infected.

97. Pest Repellent: Keep The Fleas Away.

Apple Cider Vinegar may not kill insects but its odor is pungent enough to repel insects such as bugs, flies, and even mosquitoes.

All you need do is to mix half spoon ACV and a half cup of water and put in a spray bottle to spray the furs of your pets.

Pets will stay away

98. Parasite & Bug Repelling Body Rinse.

Besides using Apple Cider Vinegar spray to repel fleas, it can be used as a rinse for repelling pests.

Into five liters of water add one cup of ACV, mix thoroughly, and use to rinse the body of your pets.

Don't let Apple Cider Vinegar get into the eyes.

Massage the solution into the body and then dry with a towel.

Do not rinse, let the solution stay on the pet's body.

I do it Kim, my Rottweiler. Other times I use Baking Soda for the same result.

You can make it a weekly bath for a better result with the fur coming out shining.

99. Pimples: Hate Them, Confidence Destroyer.

Apple Cider Vinegar will help to fight pimples but not overnight.

There is no magic here. There is nothing like getting rid of pimples overnight. You give it time to do its work over a period of time.

The organic acids in vinegar such as Acetic Acid fight the pimples and acne by killing the bacteria causing the problem. You may also get a toning effect as a bargain.

With a cotton ball, apply an equal volume of water and vinegar on the pimples. Leave for about 30 minutes and wash off. Dry up.

If you leave it overnight, no qualms, you will just get a better result.

Repeat twice a week till the pimples vanish.

I have helped a lot of people with this alone.

100. Poop (Feces Or Faeces): Clear The Bowels.

Does vinegar help you poop?

See constipation above.

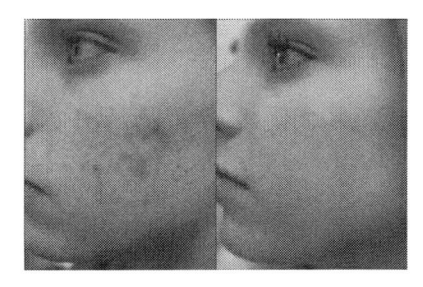

For the same reasons, Apple Cider Vinegar helps you to poop easily.

If ACV helps digestion in addition to reducing appetite and craves, it is reasonable to believe that it helps in defecating.

ACV like apples contains pectin which helps in cleaning the alimentary canal. Apple Cider Vinegar (1tablespoon) in a glass of water or use as food dressing

101. Porosity: Block The Holes.

If your hairs cuticles are opened up, you will definitely have hair porosity and you would not want to aggravate this situation by applying more heat.

What to do is invite Apple Cider Vinegar for help. It will help to close up the holes and return your hair to the normal ph.

Having washed your hair, rinse it with **ACV**

That is it. Pores are closed.

102. Healthy scalp: Home to Your Hairs.

This is what an authority on hairs said of scalp health.

"A healthy scalp is imperative to having healthy hair and fend off hair loss. Apple Cider Vinegar does help to protect your scalp by fighting off bacteria and maintaining the pH at an equilibrium level,"

We cannot argue with that, because we know Apple Cider Vinegar with all her attributes will be very useful to the scalp and its guests.

Get a spray bottle, fill it with three tablespoons of Apple Cider Vinegar, and a cup of pure water.

Spay the hair and massage the solution in, leaving it there for about fifteen minutes before you shampoo.

Your hair will thank you for the massaging which will stimulate their growth.

103. pH Balance: Balance Your Scalp PH.
See Scalp

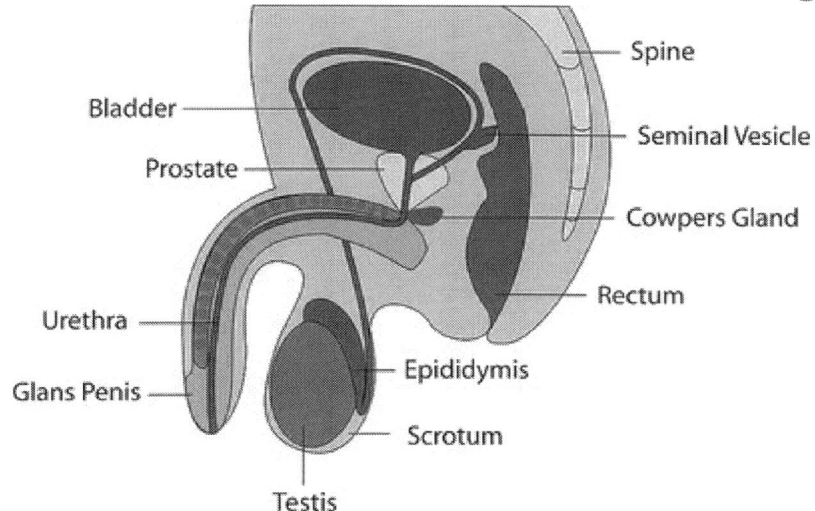

104. Prostate: Don't Allow Them to Enlarge.

Raw Apple Cider Vinegar, the unfiltered type with mother, has astringent properties that make it ideal for shrinking the prostate glands.

Do not forget, it helps weight loss and helps to prevent possible complications such as UTI (urinary Tract Infection) arising from an enlarged prostate.

Recipe.

Two tablespoons of Apple Cider Vinegar.
Two tablespoons of olive oil.
Some slices of Tomatoes.

Spice with a bit of Liquid Amino and cinnamon.

Mix together properly and use daily on Avocado, Tomatoes, and salad.

Also use Zinc, Prostex supplements which help to fight prostate.

Among the prostate fighting fruits, Tomato takes the prize.

105. Proriasis: A Smooth Skin Is The Best.

Psoriasis is a skin problem caused by a number of factors which all put pressure on the skin.

Stress, habits like smoking, and alcohol consumption can lead to Psoriasis and the result is red or silvery patches which may be accompanied by uncomfortable itches. It is common on the scalp.

There are many OTC products to treat this infection but common sense tells us that we may need to change some of the habits to get the best result.

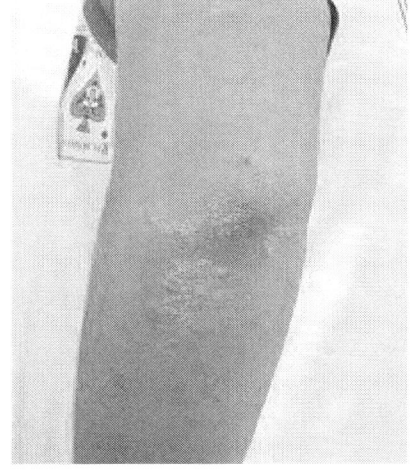

Reduce smoking and alcohol consumption.

Now, combine this with Apple Cider Vinegar treatment which does not have any side effects that one may experience from the proprietary products; you will get a good result.

1. Just apply diluted vinegar directly, sparingly on the patches several times in a week.

2. Make a fifty-fifty solution of Apple Cider Vinegar and water, soak a towel and apply directly to the affected area for about thirty minutes.

3. The Drink. One tablespoon to a cup of water. Drink daily.

106. Reflexology; Helps With Arthritis.

You could combine reflexology with Apple Cider Vinegar treatment for arthritis to get quicker relief.

See Rheumatoid Arthritis

107. Rheumatoid Arthritis: Could Be Painful.

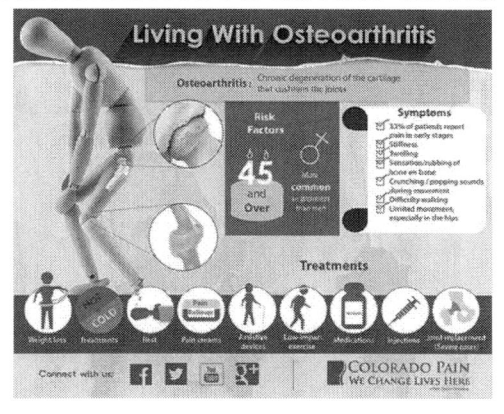

When young, we do not have acid crystals in the joints but with time and because of the junks we eat, we develop these crystals which deposit in the joints.

Before you know it, we start having tough tissues and joints leading to Arthritis and Bursitis.

If you can get a way of flushing out these acid crystals which have cemented itself with hard stony deposits in the joints, you can enjoy flexible and supple joints again.

As Apple Cider Vinegar is used in animal husbandry to soften the meat of cattle after it has been hardened by deposits of Acid crystals which make the meat tough.

Apple Cider Vinegar is equally used to soften the joints and tissue of humans, though for a different reason.

Stir a cup of distilled water with two tablespoons each of Apple Cider Vinegar and raw honey as a daily drink.

Drink plenty of pure water devoid of chemicals for soft joints

Do not forget to treat yourself to enough organic food and raw apple. Remember an apple a day, they say, keep the doctor away.

108. Scurvy.

Christopher Columbus and his men on their voyage to discover America in 1492 had barrels of vinegar for the prevention of scurvy. U.S. Civil war soldiers did the same.

So Apple Cider Vinegar had been known to fight scurvy for ages and this should be expected because it has disinfectant and healing properties.

Scurvy is caused by a lack of Vitamin C and Apple Cider Vinegar is known to have some vitamin C but not in high quantity.

You will get a better result if you eat citrus fruits with Apple Cider Vinegar treatment.

Not simultaneously, please.

Use an Apple Cider Vinegar drink.

109. Senility: Sufferers Could Be Helped.

You said what? Senile people could get real help from doses of Apple Cider Vinegar? Yes, they could.

A direct correlation has been established between senility and lack of potassium and don't forget that Apple Cider Vinegar has some quantity of potassium and also aids potassium absorption from the foods we take.

Most senile people have clogged arteries and you cannot think straight with arteries clogged with cholesterol and poison.

Potassium softens tissues just as calcium clears grimes on windows. The job of potassium is to go in and clear the arteries of the clogs.

You may not be wrong if you call potassium the body's detergent. It slows down clogging and clears clogs where they are already formed.

Organic Apple Cider Vinegar has Potassium and helps to keep tissues soft and healthy and pliable and helps to prevent heart attacks and stroke.

Two or three doses of Apple Cider Vinegar drink will not do the magic **overnight; you have to be patient with the treatment**

The Drink.

One teaspoon of ACV in a glass of water with one teaspoon of raw honey.

Drink three times a day.

Now add, multiple vitamin-mineral supplements and some niacin, vitamin B-3

Senile people could be helped. Don't write them off yet.

The above regime of Apple Cider Vinegar treatment gave a significant effect in just three weeks when applied to young children with a mental handicap.

It has similar effects on oldies as well.

See Mentally handicapped.

110.   Shampoo: Make Your Own.

It is quite simple to make shampoo at home with Apple Cider Vinegar and cheaply too leaving your hair shinning and very clean.

Get half a cup **ACV**, mix with two cups of water.

Pour the solution on your wet hair. Wash the hair with it and rinse with cold water.

You may apply using a squeeze bottle.

You may replace Apple Cider Vinegar with lemon or mix the two with water. You will get equally good results.

111.   Shingles: Chicken Pox's Sister.

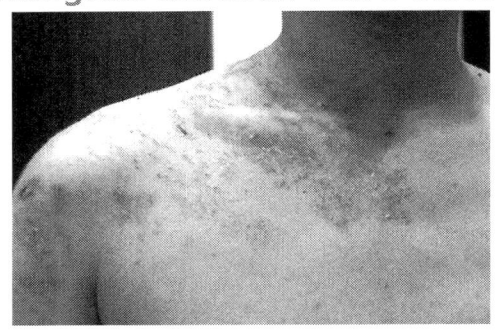

Shingle is a cluster of blisters filled with fluid around the waist often accompanied by pains and itches.

In actual fact, it could appear anywhere from the head to toe and affects more than a million people in a year.

Shingles (Heroes Zoster) a viral infection caused by reactivation of the varicella-zoster virus which could be wrestled down with Apple Cider Vinegar.

If you have had chickenpox, the virus could lie in your body and result in shingles.

Apple Cider Vinegar reduces the pain and eventually clears the rashes

Use one teaspoon of ACV to a cup of water and apply on the rashes once a day until they disappear giving you a smooth skin.

Sometimes, you have shingles in odd places like the forehead and lips. Use the same treatment.

Apple Cider Vinegar will soothe your skin and will leave it soft and supple, because It's an alpha hydroxyl compound.

The Drink. One cup of water plus one teaspoon, mix, and drink once daily. It is also good against any viral infection.

Alternatively, make a drink with one cup of green tea, a half cup of a berry e.g. strawberry, and one tablespoon of ACV.

Blend properly and drink three times a day for quick relief.

You can add two cups of ACV to the tub and have a tub birth to clear the rashes.

An equal volume of Apple Cider Vinegar and warm water could be applied with a towel to the rashes.

Variety of routes to the same destination you say.

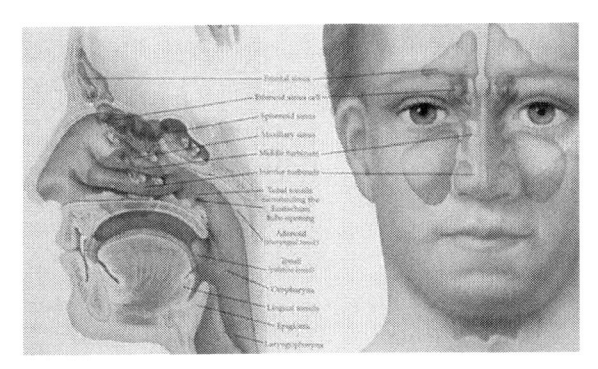

112. Sinuses : Disappears In No Time.

Sinuses are caused by microorganisms' infection and could be bacteria, viruses, or fungi.

It causes the sinus to swell giving the sufferer pains and discomfort.

The passage could be blocked producing mucus accompanied by the traditional sinus symptoms like fever, headache, pain, cough, sore throat, and nasal discharge

Breaking down mucus is one of the specialties of Apple Cider Vinegar. It follows that vinegar will drive sinuses away.

Make a cup of hot tea, add two tablespoon Apple Cider Vinegar, gulp down through the esophagus down to your stomach and experience easy breathing.

Just be sure the Apple Cider Vinegar has the 'mother' You may want to add some quantity of honey.

Steaming Treatment, remember?

One cup Apple Cider Vinegar

Four cups of hot water

Cover your head over the hot solution and breathe in the vapour.

Drink

Mix

Five parts warm water.
One-part ACV.
Plus, three tablespoons of raw honey.
Drink twice a day.

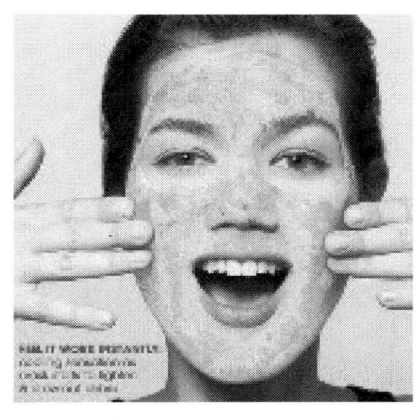

113. Skin Exfoliate: Dead Cells In Trouble.

Daily, we are bombarded with commercials urging us to make our skin lighter and succulent.

Ladies, in particular, will go to any length to have a smooth skin devoid of marks and blemishes.

To get this done, it costs some dollars here and there even with their possible side effects.

There have been cases of skin exfoliating gone wrong where skins get irreversibly damaged from the toxic chemical applications.

Apple Cider Vinegar can help to do all this without any side effects with its natural abilities.

Remember that ACV has antioxidants, minerals, and vitamins, and weak acids which are cool for the skin.

Vitamins, antioxidants, and the acids in ACV ensure exfoliating in addition to balancing the skins oil and pH for smoother skin.

Apple Cider Vinegar will remove the rashes and dead cells exposing a new glistering smooth layer of skin to the admiration of others.

Use a half cup of Apple Cider Vinegar with half a cup of water.

Apply with a towel on the face, neck, and skin. The remnant can be stored in the fridge for reuse.

With this, it will occur to you that a regular Apple Cider Vinegar tub bath will give a glower skin.

114. Sore Throat: Pharyngitis, Laryngitis Brother.

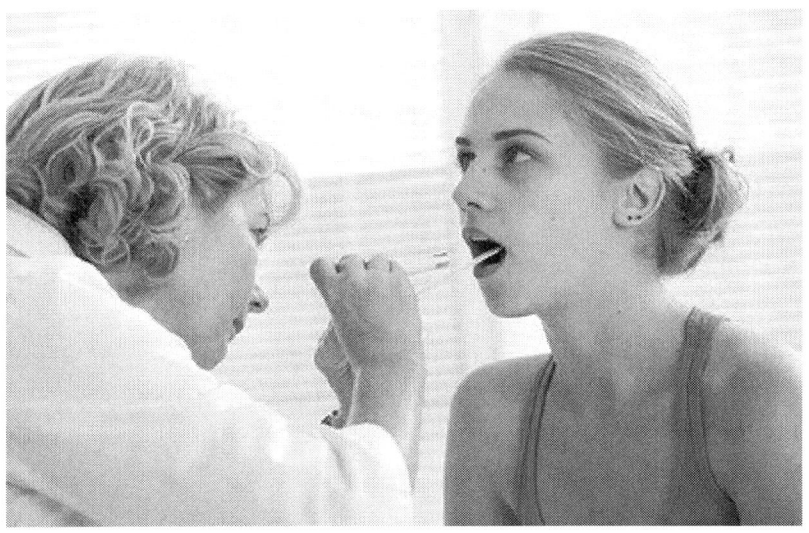

Sore throat is inflammation of the throat which is medically known as pharyngitis. It causes irritation and scratching of the throat.

It should be treated at once because it could be a precursor to more serious medical conditions.

Whether it is caused by bacteria, fungi, or viruses, raw fairly diluted Apple Cider Vinegar is well equipped to wrestle Pharyngitis to the ground.

Therapy.

A cup of warm water, one teaspoon raw honey, and one tablespoon of ACV.

You may drink the solution or gargle with it. Remember you should not swallow the gargled solution.

Laryngitis is different from Pharyngitis.

Laryngitis is the inflammation of the voice box, the larynx while Pharyngitis is the inflammation of the pharynx. The treatment is similar though.

You may want to see Laryngitis.

115. Sunburn: Summer Sun.

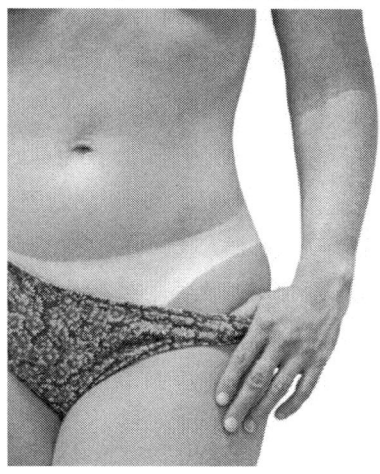

You would be right to ask why using an acidic substance like vinegar to treat sunburn but there are people who are ready to swear by Apple Cider Vinegar treatment of sunburn.

This is explainable as vinegar has antiseptic properties that kill germs in addition to reducing pain.

Just be sure you do not overdo it and if the sunburn is deep you may want to stay away from ACV so as not to aggravate the situation.

All you need do is mixing an equal volume of water and Apple Cider Vinegar and apply with cotton wool on the blisters and they will dry out.

If the sunburn is all-over, then take an ACV bath.

Pour one cup of Apple Cider Vinegar in the cool bathwater (a bucket) and enjoy the soak.

Peppermint, grated potato, and buttermilk are also good for treating sunburns.

You may want to read Burns

116. Swimmers Ear: Water in the Ear.

Swimmers ear, an infection of the outer ear can heal on its own but if it does not heal on time, antibiotics are used to treat it.

But that costs money. In its stead, you can use Apple Cider Vinegar.

You get an equal volume of ACV and warm water, not hot water, please.

Using a clean dropper bottle, apply about 5 or 6 drops in the affected ear. Get ear dropper syringe from drug stores.

Now, cover the ear with a clean cloth and rest on your side to allow the Apple Cider Vinegar solution to work in the ear.

Allow to drain out after some time.

Alternatively, you may replace warm water with rubbing alcohol (Isopropyl alcohol or diluted ethanol) This will dry the ear and fight off fungi and bacteria.

Please note that ACV can hurt your ear if used undiluted, so do not use raw Apple Cider Vinegar. Even when diluted at 1.1, it may irritate some people.

Apply a tiny drop at first and see if it irritates you. If it does, stop usage.

117. Teeth: White Teeth Give You Advantage.

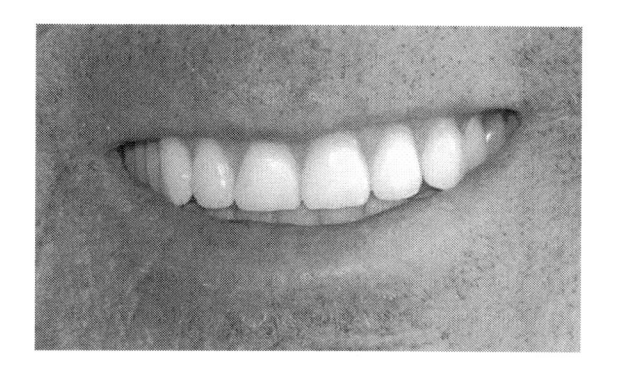

We are inundated with advertisements to make our teeth whiter.

Some in powder form, some in solutions but do they really do what they claim? Maybe, but even if they do, they don't cost peanuts.

Dentists don't charge a hundred dollars to make your teeth white. They charge in hundreds and what of the time you expend.

Those who do, have probably not heard about Apple Cider Vinegar and its numerous health uses.

As an acidic substance (weak acid) with antibacterial and antiseptic properties, it is not surprising that ACV can assist in whitening brown teeth.

The brownish color is caused by long stains and bacteria which will not stand almighty ACV.

Mix 50/50 of water, use the mouthwash to gargle the mouth thoroughly.

Spit out the gargle solution. Now use the solution to brush your teeth.

Brush the teeth normally with your normal toothpaste.

If you do this about thrice a week you should notice a significant change in the color of your teeth.

Please do not use undiluted Apple Cider Vinegar to protect the enamel of your teeth and the teeth.

118. Thirst Quencher: A Summer Need.

Do you want to quench your thirst during the summer?

Add a tablespoonful of AVC to a glass of water and a tablespoon of honey as a morning drink.

You have just taken a tonic to quench your thirst. Have a good day.

119. Thrush: A Yeast Infection.

Thrush is a yeast infection of the mouth.

See Yeast Infection.

120. Tiredness: Normal, Now Get Your Strength Back.

There are two main ways to relieve fatigue with Apple Cider Vinegar. One is through bath and the other is oral.

For bath, add about a liter of Apple Cider Vinegar into the bathwater but this may cost much.

So rub your body with Apple Cider Vinegar and take your shower bath after. Body is rejuvenated.

Your tiredness will be tired and go. You get some relief.

As for oral application. A tablespoon of Apple Cider Vinegar in a cup of water or a veg juice for you to drink will do the magic as your fatigue is reduced.

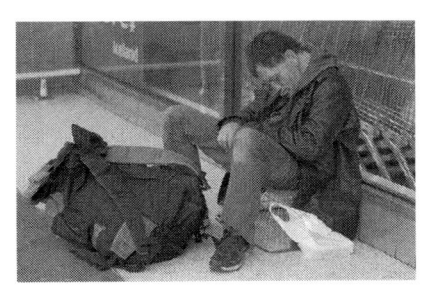

The cause of stress is the build-up of lactic acid which ACV fights with its Potassium, enzymes, and amino acids.

121. Ulcers: Don't Do It.

No, No, No.

Never, never use **Apple Cider Vinegar** for Ulcer.

For Acid reflux, Yes, For Ulcer NO.

122. Underweight: Flesh Up A Bit.

Apple Cider Vinegar is one of the greatest gifts God gave to man. It has been proving itself to be the greatest natural help to orthodox medicine.

It is natural, packed full of enzymes and other valuable compounds, and what is more, it is free of toxins.

We have said earlier that Apple Cider Vinegar fights obesity and here we are claiming it helps underweight people. Contradicting? No. not exactly.

Such is the misery of Apple Cider Vinegar. Underweight people suffer from the inability to utilize fully the food they ingest.

Here we are not talking about people who do not have enough food to it, but people who eat well and are still underweight.

No matter the quantity of fat and protein consumed they still remain underweight.

This is because they lack powerful Enzymes to convert the food to useful compounds for the body.

Deficiency of enzymes could cause weight problems.

For underweight people do an Apple Cider Vinegar cocktail for them every morning.

Two teaspoons of honey, two teaspoons of Apple Cider Vinegar in a glass of water plus two drops of Iodine from stores.

Drink this first thing in the morning.

With every meal afterward, take multi digestive enzymes.

With time such underweight people will pick up some weight.

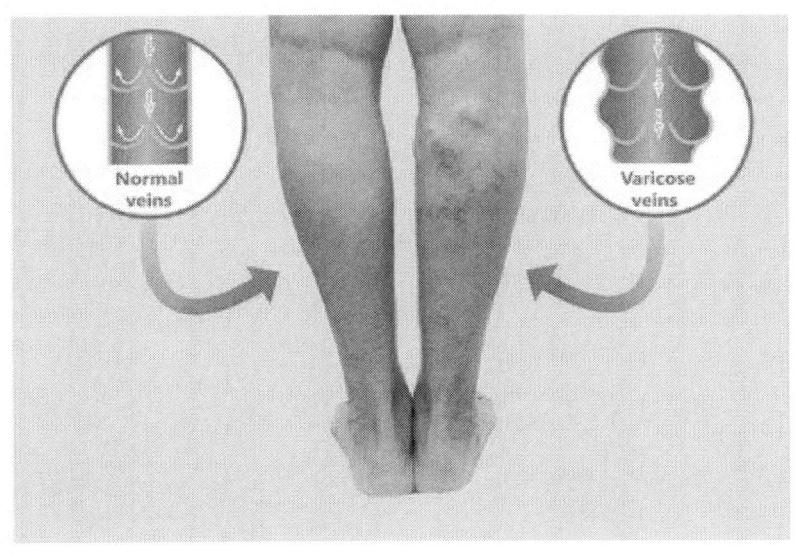

123. Varicose Veins: Ugly Sight.

When the veins of your leg, ankles, and feet especially, are colored and bulged giving an ugly sight, then know you have a varicose vein.

Often, it is caused by too much pressure on the legs or when the legs are bent at the knee. At times, it is caused by tight-fitting clothes and walking for too long.

In all cases, they lead to reduced circulation of the blood.

To get relieved, you will need to increase blood circulation to those areas. This means you will need to reverse the causes.

Do not sit down for long, do not bend your legs anyhow, and stop wearing tight dresses.

Besides the above, Apple Cider Vinegar can help.

Drinking ACV regularly will prevent those circumstances from aggravating varicose veins.

Drink.

One Tablespoon Apple Cider Vinegar.

One cup of berry e.g. strawberry.

One cup of coconut milk

Ice.

Blend properly and drink once a day.

Do you want to use Apple Cider Vinegar directly on the veins?

Dip a towel in 50/50 solution of Apple Cider Vinegar and warm water and apply on the veins for about ten minutes.

Inflammation will be reduced as blood flow will be enhanced.

124. Vegetarians And Vegans: You Need Apple Cider Vinegar.

Vegetarians and vegans in particular are not likely to get all they need from their vegetables to make the body function optimally.

Adding Apple Cider Vinegar to vegans diets will provide the ingredients to aid the absorption of micronutrients in what they consume.

This will enhance amino acid absorption and processing for better functioning of the body.

The fibres in Apple Cider Vinegar will reduce digestion issues that may be associated with plant-based food which is the bulk of a vegan food.

Apple Cider Vinegar, remember has enzymes and naturally occurring phytonutrients available in dairy products and animal protein to build immunity.

These products vegans abstain from.

Vegans will be helping themselves with a drink of one tablespoon of ACV and one cup of coconut milk or almond milk daily.

Vegetarians eat grains, fruit and vegetable eggs, and dairy products but Vegans abstain from eggs, dairy products, and any form of animal proteins.

125. Warts: No Need To Scrape.

Get a solution of one-part water and two parts Apple Cider Vinegar. Soak a cotton ball in it and place it on the wart to soften it. Bind overnight with a bandage.

Do you notice this recipe unlike others has more Apple Cider Vinegar than water? This is because we are dealing with the wart.

The strong solution will kill off the viruses and bacteria, destroys the infected skin making the skin fall off.

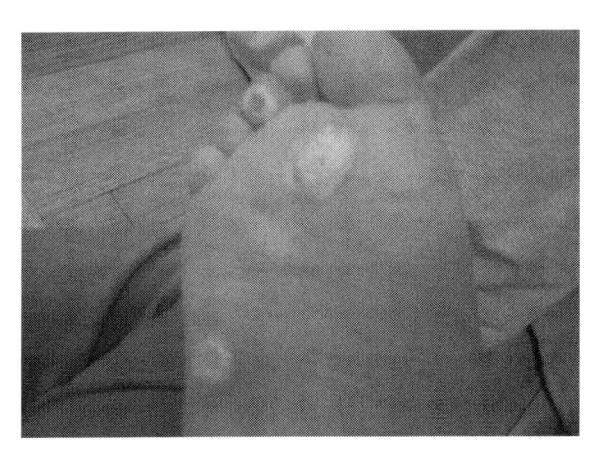

Your body's immune system is triggered to fight the virus causing the wart.

126. Weight Loss: Fat Fatty.

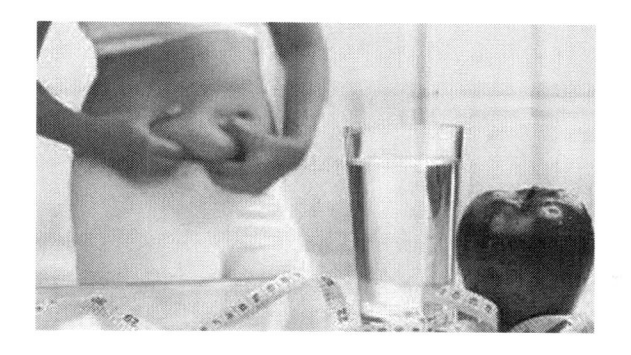

See Obesity.

127. Yeast infection.

It has been proven that Apple Cider Vinegar has both antifungal and antibacterial properties which makes it qualified to fight Candida and yeast which are caused by bacteria.

More research may be needed but we know enough to say that these fungi hate ACV.

Therefore, consuming some Apple Cider Vinegar in your meals will make your system more inhabitable for fungus and bacteria because they will not be able to thrive.

A Candida infection in the virginal is known as yeast infection which effect is drastically reduced if you douche the virginal with a mildly diluted solution of Apple Cider Vinegar with Water.

Candida infection of the mouth is referred to as thrush, which can equally be attacked with Apple Cider Vinegar mildly mixed with water.

Do the Apple Cider Vinegar gargle.

128. Yellow Nails: Make Them white.

Yellow nail is a fungal infection and if allowed to worsen, it may lead to thickening nails which may crumble with time.

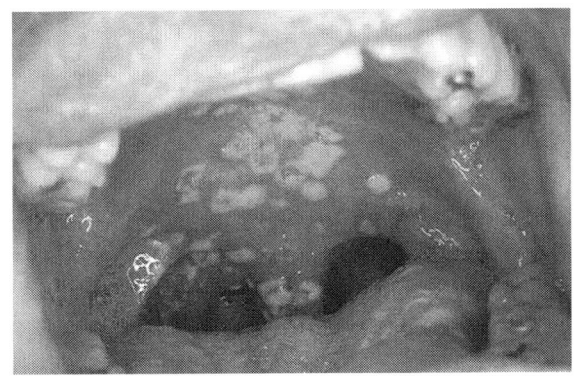

In some cases, though rare, yellow nails may be a sign of more serious medical conditions like thyroid problems, lung, diabetes, or psoriasis diseases.

You can get rid of yellow nails with Apple Cider Vinegar.

You may use white vinegar here. To one cup of warm water add one tablespoon of ACV.

Soak the nails there for ten minutes, wash and rinse your hands with warm water.

The yellow stains will disappear.

OTHER BOOKS BY THE AUTHOR.

150+ Amazing Uses Of Baking Soda You Never Knew

(Stunning Uses Of Sodium Bicarbonate In Cleaning, Beauty, Health, Organic, Home, Kitchen, Agriculture, Pesticides. Etc)

ABOUT THE AUTHOR

Richard, alternative medicine enthusiast, SME expert, and non-fiction writer hoping to have a bestseller one day. Although this is his second on Amazon, he had written three books earlier. A former teacher with a Master's degree, Richard also has experience in management and consultancy. He relaxes with friends in the evening as he believes that if you work hard; you have earned the right to spoil yourself a bit. He listens to pleasant music, engages in DIY, and enjoys playing football with his Rottweiler dog. While he uses his leg, his pet uses her teeth. Married with children who are now grown-ups, living on their own, Richard cherishes, the company of Davies, his adopted son, who makes their house sparkle and ensures their dog, Kim, has a good time.

LUCKY YOU, SO SIGN UP FOR A FREE GIVEAWAY

Click this link to grab the free gift before it expires:
www.freegift.com/secret-ebook.

WRITE A REVIEW

You may want to write a book review to share your experiences.

People will like your opinion about books you have read whether you found the books useful or not.

Giving your honest opinion about a book may help readers to know books that are ok for them.

Come back and write an honest review here.

Thanks.

ACKNOWLEDGMENT

We acknowledge the assistance of https://www.freeimages.com/ and https://www.flickr.com/ public images and Googles creative commons for the images used in this work.

Printed in Great Britain
by Amazon